GRACE

for

TROUBLED
MINDS

A MOTHER'S FAITH AND FIGHT THROUGH
THE MENTAL HEALTHCARE SYSTEM

ROSEMARIE MCCOY MCLOYD

Copyright 2019 Rosemarie McCoy McLoyd

Published by Live Limitless Authors Academy
& Publishing Co.

Contact Information
Email: limitless@sierrarainge.com
www.sierrarainge.com

Printed in the United States of America

Cover Design by Live Limitless Authors Academ.

This book is dedicated
with love to my amazing daughter Ashlee.

Ashlee, I love you!!! Since you were a little girl you have always wanted to know exactly how to do new things for yourself. I remember the first time you sat in front of the computer and I asked you to let me change the font size and colors for you. Then you asked "what is a font show me I want to do it myself" and I said okay. As I explained, you listened and said, "Okay. I got it". Then you began changing the font sizes and colors to what you wanted it to be and you had a ball with it! I love when you would read a book and always find me in the kitchen cooking dinner, and you would start telling me about the book in such an amazing way that always took me on a journey as if I was watching a movie. You have always been a great listener and worked so hard at whatever you set out to do. You have put forth extraordinary work in school and have humbly excelled in ways that your hard work is still speaking for you today. I enjoy talking to you and listening to you sing has been awesome. It is an honor watching you grow and talk about your dreams of finishing school, cooking, photography, writing your poems, completing your resume and wanting to purchase your own car yourself. It is your time of becoming an amazingly beautiful young woman of God and you will pursue and recover it all and more. You are very special to all of us Ashlee; a beautiful loving caring daughter, sister, friend and aunt. You have always looked out for other peoples' feelings. God is with you, God loves you, you're not forsaken and never forgotten. In Jesus Name!!!

Love Momma

This book is based on my personal experiences and research as I sought help for my daughter after getting a diagnosis with a mental health challenge. I first want to thank my Lord and Savior Jesus Christ for never leaving us nor forsaking us. I am grateful and thankful for all my family: my grandparents, my parents, my brother Lorenzo & his wife Marlene and my sisters Erica and Karen, and my niece Stevette. I thank my friends and my church family for their prayers, support, and encouragement to stand and not give up. I appreciate the encouragement you gave me to write and publish this book. I thank my Pastor, Dr. Riva Tims, Minister Rena` Jones, Harry Jones, Elder Michele DeCaul, Bryan DeCaul, Mother Rita Jennings, Pop Fred Jennings, Rosalynn Cook, Cassandra Brown, Caremilta Bryan, Pastor Dawn Cadle, Pastor Chauncey Brown, Marlon Woods, Gil Moffett, Michael Signil, Zachery Tims III, Genard McNeil, Lee Vayn Oliver, Deidre Council, Riccardo Hutchins, Deborah Hill, Chrystol Ingram, Katrina Wade, Nikki Boykins, William and Vanessa Adams, Tari Spear, Julissa Tabb, Giovannie Caprii, Lydell Tate, Noni Tate, Christopher Foreshaw, Al Johnson, Vernon Graham, Torrance Williams, Ed Love, Jennifer Green, Meloney Rolle, Stella Nettles, Tiffany Grant, Nina White Frazier, John Frazier, Justin Storey, Jordan Storey, Denise Myers, Kimberly Fowler, Joseph Pagan, Coleen Otero, Mo

Johnson, John Stephens, Marvin Johnson, Sandy Pollard & Cynthia Plummer.

I would like to express my special thanks of gratitude to Pastor Riva for being such a support to me and my family. I appreciate every phone call, text message, your love, and your prayers. I want to thank, my dear friend Jean Gooden for your calming strength. You are a lady of few words, however, when you speak it brings peace and order.

I want to thank my handsome son Leon Bright III for your love, support, and for being there for your sister despite your busy schedule. I want to thank my beautiful eldest daughter Shontae` and my precious grandchildren for your love and support for our family.

Thank you to my publisher Sierra Rainge-Jones for walking with me through this journey in publishing my first book. We have truly had an amazing ride. Thank you for what you do so well. I would also like to give a special thank you to my editorial angels Shontae McLoyd and Jean Gooden! Thank you for your editorial contributions and for bringing my book to life!

Thank you, GOD, for always providing and making a way out of no way, being our healer, protector; our everything!

ABOUT THE AUTHOR

By: Michele DeCaul, Elder (Majestic Life Church)

"Rosemarie McLoyd's gentle, nurturing spirit brings peace to those she comes in contact with! If she doesn't have an encouraging word to touch your heart she always has a warm delicious meal for your stomach! Her love for God makes it easy to serve and support others. Her undying commitment for her family, especially her daughter Ashlee is the driving forces behind her faith, advocacy, resourcefulness, determination, and commitment for all that she does. These qualities have allowed her to create strong relationships within her family, community, local agencies, mental health agencies, businesses, and various ministries. Her personal victories and faith in God have led her to share her heart in this book so that her encouragement and love can touch the hearts of others. She brings great strength to single mothers, parents, and families experiencing mental health challenges. Rosemarie's dedication will in no doubt leave families and the next generation with support, hope, and love! "

TABLE OF CONTENTS

Introduction

*P*arenting doesn't come with a manual. There's no guide to prepare you for the role of a lifetime. Even with all the books in the world on preparing for motherhood, or even parenting classes, there is nothing that can truly cover all the facets of motherhood. Practicing and application is a tool that is tried and true. Like most moms, when you see your baby for the first time, as you look into their new eyes, you imagine what their personalities will be like, what their voice will sound like, whose features they will inherit and what memories you can look forward to creating with them. What we never consider are the challenges that may arise on the journey and how those tough times, hardships and life changes will affect the mother and child dynamic.

My name is Rosemarie McCoy McLoyd. I am the mother of a beautiful young woman of God who has accomplished so much in her young life and still has much more to do. She and her siblings grew up very close and they looked out for one another. Her siblings are nine and twelve years older than her. She has always loved being with them. She looked up to her big sister and brother. My son went into the Navy and also attended college. My eldest daughter graduated from college as well and is now a proud mother of two children and one on the way! My son has since become a behavior therapist, he has been very instrumental in helping me with his sister. One day our lives went from 0 to 100. I went from being an orchestra mom to a full- time caregiver. I remember the day we received her first diagnosis from her doctor at the time. While waiting to speak with the doctor in order to go over details about my daughter, her history and our family, I remember feeling so anxious for an answer. I wanted to know what was wrong and more importantly how my daughter was going to get better. Can you imagine my disappointment and my frustration when the doctor finally arrived, only to come into the room to speak with us for about 5 minutes before leaving swiftly? I sat on the edge of my seat waiting for her to return to the room so that we could continue our conversation. Then, walks in a technician asking me to give consent for medications for my daughter to start taking immediately. These were medications that I had zero knowledge of and therefore I said, "No"! Clearly, I was still so unclear on what was going on. I was uninformed on her diagnosis, I was unclear about how we would move forward and how her psychosis diagnosis would affect our daily lives, and most of all I was not ready or willing to drug her up with medication when there were still so many unanswered questions. So, I requested to have a conference with the doctor for further review of the medications and to explain why she prescribed them and for what purpose. I needed to know how the medications help her, what were the possible side effects, and whether there were other treatment options.

I remember driving home with more questions than I had answers. I remember feeling overwhelmed with thought, concern, and fear if I'm speaking honestly. I was afraid that I didn't know how to fix what was wrong. I so desperately wanted clarity; I needed a solution. In my community, African American women of faith typically handle mental health issues with a prayer request or an altar call. While I put all my trust in God, I wanted to offer my daughter all the support available to her. Even with a powerful village of prayer warriors pleading to heaven on our behalf for healing, I felt compelled to subscribe to professional help as well. I couldn't help but feel like my daughter needed both.

That drive home felt so lonely. I knew that I had a church community and even family who loved us and would be supportive, but the truth is, I didn't know anyone else who was dealing with a mental health crisis. I had no one to call who could really understand what it was like to become an overnight, full-time caretaker for a teenager who was once completely fine and is now suffering from a mental health crisis. I questioned, who will understand? Who would spare judgment? Who will offer guidance?

Today I feel empowered and hopeful. I have become more educated on my daughter's diagnosis and I've learned to effectively manage our lives. I've been able to adjust so that my daughter always feels safe and supported. Just as important, I've learned just how critical it is to prioritize self-care as a caregiver.

If you're reading this book, you or someone you love has been diagnosed with a mental health condition. You may be looking for tools to help you cope with or better understand how to adjust, you may want resources to help you make informed decisions about your treatment plan, or maybe you need faith-based daily devotions that offer insight that will compel you to extend grace during moments of trouble. I wrote this book with you in mind. Our country is suffering from a mental health crisis. There is a great need to increase awareness and counter negative stigma with compassion, understanding, and knowledge.

I know that there is a need to overcome religious barriers that prevent individuals from seeking treatment and professional help. To effect change in this area, I started a mental health and disability Ministry called 'Never Walking Alone' at my church, *Majestic Life Church*, with the support of my pastor Dr. Riva Tims, along with other leaders and volunteers.

My goal is to help families, individuals and professionals know that the stigmas that are attached to mental health and disabilities have to be shut down. Shame causes families and individuals to suffer in silence! I am not ashamed of this journey that I'm walking with my daughter and my goal is to help other parents, mothers, fathers, and siblings to stand beside their loved ones and say, "I am not ashamed". Most of all, I want people to know that just because something is happening with your child does not mean that something is wrong with you.

Most of the time when your loved one is stricken with a mental health disorder; people immediately retreat to isolation and shame because we don't want anyone to think that something is wrong with us. Well, we must change our mindset on how we look at mental health and disabilities. Take, for example, the way we should look at a broken arm.

If someone in your family had a broken arm you would not sit silently. You would take them to the doctor. If you had a broken arm you would not sit silently, you would also go to the doctor. We have to be just as proactive when it comes to ailments of the mind. It's okay to get help, we all process things differently in this life! When traumatic things happen, the way you process it may be different than your neighbor or the way the person across the street will process it and within that process things happen. Triggers happen and so we must look at the whole person and not just the symptoms of what you're seeing on the outside. Show people compassion and love the same love that you would want someone to show you. Therefore, my goal, with the help of the Lord, is to shut down the stigmas that are attached with mental illness and disabilities. Shame causes isolation which can lead to suicide. I will continue to move forward in this journey with my daughter because the Lord has taught me in this process through His word (Romans 5:5) "that in the midst of my troubles, hope maketh not ashamed". So, because of hope in my Lord and Savior Jesus Christ, I know that there is a victory on the other side of this for her and for others in Jesus mighty name.

There is work to be done and more resources are needed to help give a better quality of health care services and everyday living for those who are walking this journey.

From Emotional Pain in Brain for First Time

By Maia Szalavitz @maiasz May 06, 2013

New research suggests physical pain may have a distinct brain "signature" that distinguishes it from emotional hurt. In the brain, the pain from broken leg and the anguish of a broken heart share much of the same circuitry. But the latest evidence points to distinct ways that the brain processes each type of pain and could lead to a greater understanding of how to detect and treat them.

FAMILY DYNAMICS

The word family came into English in the fifteenth century. Its roots lie in the Latin word *famulus*, which means "servant". The first meaning in English was close to our modern word "household"; defined as a group of individuals living under one roof which included blood relatives and servants.

In one day, my life changed completely. In fact, the lives of my entire family changed completely. We had to learn a new way of living. It is difficult to find the words to describe what that felt like, but let me take a moment to try. Looking back, I realize that the change didn't, in fact, happen in one day. It was a series of events that seemed to have reached a breaking point one day, and from that day on, our lives have not been the same.

It started when my husband and I separated, and then amplified when we later divorced. Slowly what was taking root in our family was abandonment and rejection. There are a lot of divorces in our western culture and even more around the world. The divorce itself is hard to deal with because it takes on a form of grief that can mirror the loss experienced through death. If there's one thing I can share with parents, it's that when a couple makes a decision that they no longer want to be together, it's important to consider the fact that you're not only affecting one another; but divorce affects your children too. A lot of times, children are trying to find out if it's something that they have done wrong that has caused the family to split. They often wonder if there was something they could have done to make their parents stay together. They may not say these things to you, but you would be surprised at how much children internalize from a divorce. They have to come to terms with the idea of their parents living separate lives, they have to process what life is like now that their parents have broken up. Even if it wasn't the best family, it was the only family they knew. Let's face it, there is nothing good about the word divorce.

I believe in the sanctity of marriage. I did not get married with the intent of getting divorced. I was 19 years old when I met my ex-husband and we were married for 27 years. I often thought about us growing old together and playing with our grandchildren. However, that is not what happened. Divorce dramatically changed our family dynamic. It affected our family emotionally. Emotional pain can take on the characteristics of physical pain, which can then cause triggers and illnesses; both mental and physical.

It's imperative that fathers understand just how much their daughters need them. Fathers are needed, the role they play in the lives of their sons and daughters is invaluable. It takes a man to raise another man, and daughters want to be adored by their fathers. So, when you've made the decision to move forward in your life, and you decide that divorce is the best option … don't divorce your children. Find a healthy way to co-parent. Mothers and fathers must find a way to communicate better and to find a way to move forward in peace and in harmony by always putting the children first.

I don't have all of the answers because I really would like to take the word divorce off the table, however, we know that there are many families who live in the state of divorce. Communicating with your children is so important and staying present in their lives is so necessary. Find the balance between no longer living in the same household.

Statistics show that the divorce rate is still high in the U.S. at 53%. Additionally, Spain, Portugal, Luxembourg, the Czech Republic, and Hungary are worse off with divorce rates higher than 60%.

Belgium has the highest rate of divorce in this data set at a staggering 70%. The lowest official rate is in Chile with 3%.

These alarmingly high instances of divorce contribute to the prevalence of life dissatisfaction and ultimately depression, anxiety, and other forms of mental illness.

When divorce causes trauma in the family and it affects one of your loved ones, rally around them as a family and show them all the love that you can possibly show them. Extend them grace to ease their troubled mind. As you seek out resources and professional services, be sure to seek and trust God. I pray all the time for wisdom and guidance. I asked God to give me insight and to teach me how to go about helping my daughter through her mental health crisis. I also prayed for resources.

It's key that your loved one feels supported. Be there for them and always try to surround them with those who have their best interest at heart. Placing them in the right environment with the right people can help bring comfort during a tough time.

Never stop living! It may not be easy, in fact, I guarantee you it won't be easy. There will be some challenging times but do not give up because you are more than conquerors through Christ Jesus. My hope is that you will find some comfort in my words and know that it will get better, even if what your loved one is going through doesn't change right away. Through the process, there's so much that is taking place. Walk through this journey one step at a time, one day at a time, one moment at a time, one second at a time and I promise you that God is already working it out. He is making provisions. There were days when I could not leave my apartment because I was there with my daughter and she wasn't in a mental state that allowed her to be left home alone. There was a season when I couldn't go anywhere, and thankfully that has changed. I got to the point where I truly had to trust God and He showed me that I can trust Him and know that everything is going to be alright.

In those moments and days when I could not leave my apartment, I found myself in a state of frustration and loneliness. When I got into the word of God and I began to speak life into the atmosphere, my environment and my mindset began to change. I began to experience growth from the inside out. I no longer felt the frustration and I no longer felt alone. So, when you start to feel alone and you're feeling frustrated, I highly recommend that you pick up your bible and begin to read it. Even if you've never read the bible before, pick it up and start reading it in your atmosphere and watch things begin to change for you.

There was a time when I had to schedule everything around my son's timeline for me to go anywhere or handle business. I had to wait until my son was able to be with my daughter based on his work schedule. Thus, we worked around each other's schedules so that we could always have that support for her. We've been very determined to have her at home with family to show her love and support. My son also accompanied me to most of my daughter's doctor's appointments as well. Was it challenging? Yes, however when faced with a challenge that's another opportunity for God to show you His love and power in your life.

GRACE FOR TROUBLED MINDS

Repeat the Lord's prayer during moments of heaviness. This prayer brings comfort because it's a reminder that God is with you, even during hard times.

Matthew 6: 9-13 New King James Version (NKJV)

[9] After this manner therefore pray ye: Our Father which art in heaven, Hallowed be thy name.

[10] Thy kingdom come, Thy will be done in earth, as it is in heaven.

[11] Give us this day our daily bread.

[12] And forgive us our debts, as we forgive our debtors.

[13] And lead us not into temptation, but deliver us from evil: For thine is the kingdom, and the power, and the glory, forever. Amen.

NOTES:

REMOVING THE C WORD

For far too long, society has marginalized and ostracized those who suffer from mental health conditions. There is an overwhelming level of intolerance for those who live with mental challenges if you don't believe me, just consider the homeless demographic in your community. Mental illness is one of the greatest contributors to homelessness. We must move toward a level of consciousness that gives mental ailments the same merit and compassion of physical illness. When someone suffers from cancer or diabetes, they are never considered crazy or looked down upon. Unfortunately, the same is not true for those with disorders of the mind. The negative stigmas that are associated with mental health is a barrier to treatment. Individuals are less likely to seek professional help because they fear to have to wear the "C" label. So, if you love someone who is suffering from mental anguish, confusion, anxiety, depression or one of the many forms of mental illness, do us all a favor, don't call them "crazy". The negative effects of using the word crazy are detrimental on so many levels. When you look at the different definitions of the word crazy, it can also mean that someone is extremely enthusiastic about another person, passionate, fanatical and excited about something. Then on the other hand, when you hear someone you love being called crazy when they are having challenges in their mind, it takes on a whole different meaning; a whole different point of view for the person whom you know to be an amazing and loving individual. The word "crazy" is deplorable and demeaning. When someone is going through something in their mind that has been caused by triggers from life events, it could be someone you love, a neighbor or the person across the street.

A stranger who was living a normal everyday life going to work, going to school and one day something happened. It could have been a physical injury; it could have been an emotional trauma or maybe even divorce in the family. Now, this person is no longer responding to life as usual. We see the symptoms and one of the first things people say is they're "crazy". When you think about it that's really sad of us as a society, because this can happen to anyone at any given moment. We all process things differently in life. I would say that we need to stop calling individuals "crazy". I challenge you to look deeper than what you see on the surface. Don't call them what they do, don't call them the assumed symptoms that you see. Call them who they are, call them by name. Call them the best of who they are when they're at their worst. That will cause them to rise above what is happening. When someone is going through a tough time, use your words to speak healing and comfort. When you use your words to comfort someone who is feeling down or depressed, you give them strength and hope to heal. Speaking positive words can help them to start to see themselves changing inside out. Then what is happening around them will begin to change. For example, if you have a child that's acting out and if you continue to call that child bad, that child is going to continue to show you exactly what you're calling them. On the other hand, if you sit that child down and begin to talk to them about who they are and the good things that you see in them as opposed to the symptoms and their perceived negative actions, you remind them of the good in them. People are much more than their circumstances. Apostle Paul in Romans 7 verse 15 through 20.

"I do not understand what I do, for what I want to do, I do not do, but what I hate I do and if I do what I do not want to do I agree that the law is good as it is no longer I myself what do it but it is sin living in me for I know that good itself does not dwell in me that is in my sinful nature for I have a desire to do what is good but I cannot carry it out for I do not do the good I want to do but the evil I do not want to do this I keep on doing not if I do what I do not want to do it is no longer I who do it but it is sin living in me that does it."

Now you may be asking: Why did the author use this example? Paul who was an apostle of Jesus Christ, in his sound mind, explaining here in scripture that even he had challenges doing what was right and that he would desire not to make the right choices. Consequently, because of sin in the flesh, he does it anyway. Thus, what Paul is saying is that "this thing that you see I have done is not who I am". Equivalently, when someone is going through a traumatic time in their life, how and why do we choose to call them "crazy"? It must change, we must choose to call them who they are and remind them of the person that you know them to be. Call them who God says they are. The more you call them who they really are, you will begin to see them demonstrate who they really are and cause them to rise above what's happening. Don't push them deeper into the quicksand by labeling and shaming them.

The "C" word itself is used too loosely and too often at the wrong times. It is very insensitive, and it does not make anyone feel better especially if they're going through something in their mind. Just pause for a moment and think about what you speak before you say it. Do your very best to always lean towards speaking the most positive words into someone else's life. I can give you an example: While I was going through some challenges trying to get help for my daughter, my pastor Dr. Riva Tims, ministers in my church, friends, and family all spoke positive words into my life at a time when I was at my lowest. They were speaking so much positivity into my life, it caused me to rise above my despair and it was also breaking the negativity off my mind. I was able to step into the greatness of who I am and tower through every obstacle and every challenge that I faced trying to get resources for my daughter. Through the word of God, it brings positivity to your mind body and soul. In my research, I found that the brain registers pain the same no matter where it comes from. For example, if you stomp your toe or if someone hurts your feelings it all registers the same in the brain. Emotional pain takes on the same characteristics as physical pain. When someone hurts your feelings, you may feel pain in your stomach, get a headache or feel nauseous. Negative words bring on emotional pain which leads to physical pain which leads to illness in the body and mental trauma.

Positive words do the total opposite. It causes someone to rise, to be triumphant, to overcome, be set free, experience release, to accelerate, to catapult, to gain upward momentum and move forward into the greatness of who they're purposed to be!

We must get serious about normalizing mental health treatment starting on our jobs. We need to be more informed and intentional when we select our healthcare, dental and vision care packages. Mental health should have its own section as an election for services. A lot of plans have mental health coverage and most people are unaware of it. We have to take the shock and shame out of talking about mental health and disabilities. It should be a part of our day-to-day conversation, in church, on our jobs, grocery shopping, our dinner tables, etc. We should be able to recommend resources, just as we recommend a dentist. For every visit to the doctor, there should be a mental health checkup. Let's talk about why patients and individuals shy away from these types of conversations especially in the doctor's office. We have to make the conversation less intimidating. Patients are in fear that someone is going to try to institutionalize them. By working together to normalize mental health in our communities, together we will shut down the shame and fear. Just like we have an HOA and a neighborhood watch in our communities, we should create a system within our communities for mental health and disabilities awareness for support.

There needs to be an increase in training, a call for more volunteers and more support for families. We have to train more crisis intervention officers and first responders across the country to recognize the symptoms and get the right help. The role of crisis intervention teams in policing communities. These situations can be tense and often misinterpreted, but having the proper training for officers responding to these calls can help them to recognize when individuals are suffering from a mental health crisis. The lack of mental health crisis services across the U.S. have resulted in law enforcement officers serving as first responders. A Crisis Intervention Team (CIT) program is an innovative, community-based approach to improve the outcomes of these encounters.

Statement from | NAMI: National Alliance on Mental Illness ●

Grace for troubled minds: Focus on your Faith

"Fight the good fight of faith. Take hold of the eternal life to which you were called when you made your good confession in the presence of many witness" **1 Tim. 6:12**

This scripture inspires us to remember who we are. It allows us to see ourselves the way that God sees us. It's a fresh perspective. God perceives us as whole and complete, healed and in alignment with what His word says about us.

REFLECT AND JOURNAL YOUR THOUGHTS.

_____

_____

_____

_____

_____

_____

_____

_____

_____

_____

_____

_____

_____

_____

_____

_____

_____

Daily Devotion:

Proverbs 3 King James Version (KJV) 3 "My son, forget not my law; but let thine heart keep my commandments: 2 For length of days, and long life, and peace, shall they add to thee. 3 Let not mercy and truth forsake thee: bind them about thy neck; write them upon the table of thine heart: 4 So shalt thou find favor and good understanding in the sight of God and man. 5 Trust in the Lord with all thine heart; and lean not unto thine own understanding. 6 In all thy ways acknowledge him, and he shall direct thy paths. 7 Be not wise in thine own eyes: fear the Lord, and depart from evil. 8 It shall be health to thy navel, and marrow to thy bones. 9 Honor the Lord with thy substance, and with the first fruits of all thine increase: 10 So shall thy barns be filled with plenty, and thy presses shall burst out with new wine. 11 My son, despise not the chastening of the Lord; neither be weary of his correction: 12 For whom the Lord loveth he correcteth; even as a father the son in whom he delighteth. 13 Happy is the man that findeth wisdom, and the man that getteth understanding. 14 For the merchandise of it is better than the merchandise of silver, and the gain thereof than fine gold. 15 She is more precious than rubies: and all the things thou canst desire are not to be compared unto her. 16 Length of days is in her right hand; and in her left-hand riches and honor. 17 Her ways are ways of pleasantness, and all her paths are peace. 18 She is a tree of life to them that lay hold upon her: and happy is every one that retaineth her. 19 The Lord by wisdom hath founded the earth; by understanding hath he established the heavens. 20 By his knowledge the depths are broken up, and the clouds drop down the dew. 21 My son, let not them depart from thine eyes: keep sound wisdom and discretion: 22 So shall they be life unto thy soul, and grace to thy neck. 23 Then shalt thou walk in thy way safely, and thy foot shall not stumble. 24 When thou liest down, thou shalt not be afraid: yea, thou shalt lie down, and thy sleep shall be sweet. 25 Be not afraid of sudden fear, neither of the desolation of the wicked, when it cometh. 26 For the Lord shall be thy confidence, and shall keep thy foot from being taken. 27 Withhold not good from them to whom it is due, when it is in the power of thine hand to do it. 28 Say not unto thy neighbor, Go, and come again, and tomorrow I will give; when thou hast it by thee. 29 Devise not evil against thy neighbor, seeing he dwelleth securely by thee. 30 Strive not with a man without cause, if he has done thee no harm. 31 Envy thou not the oppressor, and choose none of his ways. 32 For the forward is abomination to the Lord: but his secret is with the righteous. 33 The curse of the Lord is in the house of the wicked: but he blesseth the habitation of the just. 34

Surely, he corneth the scorners: but he giveth grace unto the lowly. 35 The wise shall inherit glory: but shame shall be the promotion of fools.

Understanding
Diagnosis

I wasn't given the opportunity to understand the diagnosis in the beginning. It seemed as if the doctors were moving forward with treatment and weren't adequately helping me understand what exactly we were treating. Once my daughter was admitted to the hospital and I answered a few questions. I waited for the doctor to come into the room and I waited anxiously to have a conversation with her to find out more about what was happening. She talked to me for about five minutes, she then left the room. Shortly after, another technician came into the room and she gave me medications to approve for my daughter. I looked at her and I said, "I'm waiting for the doctor to come back. She was only in here for about five minutes, is she coming back?" The technician responded, "Ma'am, No! She's gone, she's already with another patient. They wanted me to authorize medications". I looked at her, and I said, "No, I want to talk to her, I want to know more about what's happening. I don't understand what's going on". This was my first experience with understanding the diagnosis. I asked the doctor to call me to talk to me. I wanted her to give me more of an explanation as to why she prescribed these particular medications. I had another conversation with the doctor, and I agreed to the first treatment and to the medications. I was very nervous because I read the side effects. It was unknown territory for me. At this point, I still lacked a full understanding of what was going on with my daughter. My primary thing was I just wanted her to be safe. I visited her with family and friends. I continued to talk to the doctors and the main thing that they talked about were the symptoms that they were seeing outwardly. I started to do my own research online to find out if there were exams that could be given to her; the psychiatric hospitals don't perform many screenings. Furthermore, I wanted to know if other doctors could be brought in for a second opinion or for additional support, but they don't collaborate with other doctors like a neurologist while they're inside of the hospital. The diagnosis they gave me was psychosis (NOS); not otherwise specified. I am still in the process of understanding the diagnosis. I feel that if the mental health community of doctors would collaborate, more patients would get a more well-rounded perspective on treatment options.

Throughout my daughter's hospitalizations, I have been her advocate. Therefore, being an advocate and a mom who loves her daughter, I continue to do my research for every medication treatment suggested by the doctors for my daughter. I have done research on the diagnosis and I continue to advocate for her to get better care and to get the authorizations for her to see other doctors. I pray for my daughter every day I pray for clear direction concerning medications and side effects. She's more than a diagnosis, she's more than these medications, she's more than the symptoms that you see. There's so much more to her, so much more living for her to do.

With the way mental health is being addressed in today's healthcare system, you must become an advocate for health awareness. Prepare for meetings with your doctor by writing out a list of questions, concerns, and symptoms. Ask the doctor to provide literature and resources that you can read to gain more knowledge. Don't be afraid to get a second opinion.

My daughter was experiencing adverse effects from her prescribed medications and a well-known hospital was recommended for me to take her to. The hospital was about three hours from where we lived. With the support of family members, we drove her to the hospital. It was difficult to leave her there because it was so far from home. Before leaving, we all held hands and she led us in prayer. A few days later, the hospitals had a court hearing. It is a part of their procedure to determine how long individuals will be hospitalized. There were several doctors and there was also a doctor to give a second opinion.

During the hearing, one of the doctors suggested that my daughter be recommended for a state hospital because she was "loud", these were the doctor's exact words. During that hearing, as I sat there quietly due to the strict court rules that prohibited interruptions when I heard what that doctor said my stomach sank. At this point in time, I had no knowledge about state hospitals, but as soon as they mentioned it something went through my entire body. There were bells going off like something is not right. I only brought her there to have her medications adjusted and to have testing done. My goal was for her to come back home. She had been doing so well up until her prolonged exposure to the prescribed medications.

Unfortunately, most doctors have told me that it's trial and error when it comes to prescribing medication. As I sat there listening, I began to pray and ask God to give me the strength to remain calm. My prayer was that when I began to speak, they would hear me and not just see me.

When I started to talk, I began by telling them who my daughter was and not what they were seeing. My daughter had recently had a beautiful birthday party. I was able to give her a beautiful party where she was on the stage singing and she was still doing the day-to-day things like singing in our choir. I described to them how her behavior started to change after being on the medications for a while. This is why I brought her there in the first place. I let them know that I expected for her to come home because we did have support and people praying for us.

After I finished speaking, they asked me to go into a room to watch a video and they told me that someone would be joining me, and I could not speak to this person. I am an adult, yet I was instructed not to speak or talk to the person in the room with me. That person was in training and they were evaluating the same procedure that they were asking me to evaluate. When the person entered the room, I saw that it was the same person that was sitting in the hearing. Mind you, I didn't say anything to the person however the person started speaking to me and this is what she said, "Ms. McLoyd, when you began to speak about your daughter, I heard every word. Your daughter is so blessed to have you and I wish you the best with everything that you're trying to do for her". Then I expressed my gratitude for her kind and encouraging words.

I continued watching the video, now the video that they wanted me to watch was a procedure that they wanted to perform on my daughter. That procedure is called ECT (electronic shock therapy) They asked me to go and do my own research.

When I left the room, several nurses approached me and asked me would I be giving them permission to start it right away. "No!", I told them. I wanted to be very prayerful and to do my due diligence in research. I let the nurse that I would be in touch with my decision. I had a three-hour drive home. I was driving and praying. I began to get instructions on how to do my research, they told me to look up ECT. The Holy Spirit began to minister to me to look up ECT and the heart because at the time my daughter was dealing with tachycardia. During the follow-up appointment, I informed them of her condition when I discovered that they were not giving her the medication for tachycardia.

When you look up ECT and the heart muscle, you will find a lot more information versus looking at ECT by itself. With my findings, I was able to go back to the doctor with a witness present as he and I talked. I asked the doctor how he planned to treat a patient with tachycardia when it comes to ECT. He said, "well that's a good question". I responded, "because I have shared with the staff that my daughter is dealing with a heart condition and they have not been giving her the medication". I let him know that I found out in my research that the ECT causes the heart rate to spike, and if you're already dealing with a rapid heart rate it could be problematic. I asked him how he planned to handle that and he again said, "that's a good question"

The witness and I sat waiting for answers, the doctor asked me to give him a few minutes. He then went to retrieve my daughter's chart. After some delay and a few more rounds, the doctor let me know that he would be in touch with me regarding my concerns. We were about fifteen minutes into the drive back home when I got a phone call. The doctor stated, "Ms. McLoyd, I want to start by saying that we're very lucky to have you working with us to help us with your daughter's care". He then proceeded to say, "your daughter is not a candidate for ECT". He then told me that he would also put in place the other things that I had requested. He started her back on the medications for tachycardia immediately. We talked about her length of stay and what my concerns were based on what was said in the hearing, so once I got home, I continued to pray and again the Holy Spirit began to minister to me and give me strategies.

I printed off all the pictures of all the activities and everything my daughter had recently been doing with her in-home therapist. I packaged them in a confidential envelope and gave them to the doctor to show him the things that she can do and the things that she had been doing. I only brought her there to get better treatment and to check her medications. I wanted to get help for her, I wanted a better regiment, and for them to do more testing. The testing that I requested was not done because Medicaid did not cover it.

My daughter had not done anything to anyone there, except try to help other people by praying for them. Unfortunately, because she would get loud, a doctor wanted to send her to a state hospital. I went home and began my research about state hospitals here in my state. I found horrifying information. Most of the Florida State facilities are inhumane, deplorable, understaffed, and unsafe. I even called newspapers to talk to the reporters who wrote some of the articles that I read. Throughout this entire horrifying experience, I kept my focus on GOD. I stayed in prayer and waited for instructions from the Lord. The WORD of God says, "He will lead us and guide us!" I am a living witness.

After the doctor looked at the photos that I had left for him, he called me the next day and stated that my daughter was doing so much better and that there were never any incidents reported. She was compliant with taking her medications, then he said that he was amazed by what he saw in the photographs. He then asked me what time I wanted to pick her up. I picked her up the next day and brought back home.

Now, Look at GOD!

Each year, about 5,000 Floridians are sent to one of the state's seven mental health facilities. Some have been committed under the Baker Act for evaluation and treatment.

By law, the state has a duty to treat those patients with dignity and respect. But a new audit reveals several serious shortcomings within Florida's mental health institutions: The facilities are understaffed, unlicensed, and don't meet building or fire codes.

Staff at the seven facilities failed to complete incident reports as required. In four cases, including two suicide attempts and two verified instances of abuse or neglect, employees waited more than 24 hours before contacting the state facilities director.

(Lipscomb, 2017)

Recognizing Triggers

What is a trigger might you ask?

Trigger | Definition of Trigger by
Merriam-Webster › dictionary › trigger

1: to initiate, actuate, or set off by a trigger an indiscreet remark that triggered a fight a stimulus that triggered a reflex.

I thought it was important to start with the definition so that you understand that the words and actions you take can trigger something that is lying dormant in another individual. This could cause them to have a mental shift in their mindset without you ever knowing it. It doesn't always mean that the individual has a mental illness; however, it can cause them to shut down or to have a break in reality because of something that may have happened in their childhood or something that could have happened yesterday.

There's no way for you to really know just by looking at an individual; however, we should be very mindful of the words that we use or the actions that we take. A trigger for someone could be a song on the radio, changes in the seasons, cologne, foods, smells or colors.

When you think of someone who joins the military, because of the experiences in the military, they now suffer from PTSD. The sound of a firecracker could bring back memories of the battlefield. Posttraumatic stress disorder (PTSD) is a psychiatric disorder that can occur in people who have experienced or witnessed a traumatic event such as a natural disaster, a serious accident, a terrorist act, war/combat or other acts of violence.

Understanding that a physical injury can cause mental trauma and mental trauma can bring on physical illnesses. Some physical traumas; such as a head injury may mimic mental illnesses. If you see your loved one acting differently after a head injury; get the proper testing done. Seek help right away, our mindset is so critical to our wellness. Someone can speak a word and send you into a downward spiral. You have the power to not allow it to affect you, by remaining calm and staying positive. Emotional pain will try to replay in your mind over and over. Emotional pain is something that you're able to feel as if it just happened. However, physical pain depending on the degree of the injury; you won't even think about it and you cannot duplicate that same level of pain in your mind. How does the brain process pain? The same part of the brain *temporal lobe* - the anterior insula and cingulate cortex, responds to physical pain and emotional pain. The parietal lobe is also involved in interpreting pain and touch in the body.

By understanding how the brain works, with the help of GOD, you have the power to shut down the negativity. By fueling your mind with positive words, the word of GOD, positive thinking will change your outlook and shift your mindset.

For example, you wake up in a great mood, excited about your day and out of nowhere a feeling comes over you. You're now feeling sad and you notice that your mood is changing. The first thing you should do is focus on where you're feeling the change the most. Start with the physical aspects of it. For example, you may be experiencing stomach pain, a headache, arm ache, pain in your leg or back. More than likely a thought came to you. That's usually the number one source. Other things could be a phone call, a song on the radio or a subtle comment. It could be several things. You get the point I'm making.

Pay close attention to things like this and especially changes in seasons. This one is big; it's very subtle. You may notice your loved one or friend acting the same way around the same time of the year. Changes in their mood, withdrawal from family and friends. It may be because of something that may have happened years ago or may have just recently happened. Triggers are common and it could be you one day; no one is exempt from the experience of triggers.

I am sharing this information to help you recognize when your mood is changing and how you have the power to overcome it. Also, to help you recognize triggers that you may see in your loved ones, friends or a stranger. You can better help them by being more aware and having knowledge.

Recognizing it is the first step. Seek help from your church or a professional. It's okay to make these types of conversation a fixture of your everyday conversations. This will help others to not suffer in silence and more likely to ask for help. Find a healthy yet sensitive way to start the talk.

Take a moment to think about moments in your life where you may have been triggered by something. What triggered you? What memories were brought forth from your subconscious?

_____

_____

_____

_____

_____

_____

_____

_____

_____

Before I conclude this chapter, I would like to touch on the topic of forgiveness. It is vital and very important in the healing process. Forgiveness of others and yourself. Ask for help, I pray that you find some comfort and peace through the WORD OF GOD. Find peace in the scriptures below.

1. "…I am the Lord who heals you." (Exodus 15:26)- (GOD IS A HEALER THROUGH HIS SON JESUS CHRIST).

2. "I will restore you to health and heal your wounds 'declares the Lord…" (Jeremiah 30:17) (BELIEVE THE PROMISES OF GOD OVER YOUR LIFE-SEE YOURSELF HEALED, WHOLE AND SET FREE).

3. "As a mother comforts her child, so I will comfort you; …" (Isaiah 66:13) (LATE IN THE

MIDNIGHT HOUR GOD IS GOING TO TURN IT AROUND - HE WILL NEVER LEAVE YOU NOR FORSAKE YOU).

4. "…Jesus graciously welcomed them and talked to them about the kingdom of God. Those who needed healing, he healed." (Luke 9:10-11) (BY HIS STRIPES YOU ARE HEALED).

5. "Lord, you know how I long for my health once more. You hear my every sigh." (Psalm 38:9) (GOD SEES YOUR TEARS AND HEARS YOUR CRIES AND HE SHALL DELIVER YOU).

6. "Yes, I will bless the Lord and not forget the glorious things he does for me. He forgives all my sins. He heals me." (Psalm 103:2) (HALLELUJAH THANK YOU GOD FOR YOUR LOVE, YOUR HEALING POWER OVER MY LIFE AND THE LIVES OF MY FAMILY- THANK YOU FOR MANIFESTING YOUR PROMISES IN MY LIFE- FOR YOUR GLORY LORD - IN JESUS NAME- AMEN. I BELIEVE!).

7. "Beloved, I wish above all things that thou mayest prosper and be in health, even as thy soul prospereth." (3 John 2) (WE SERVE A

WONDERFUL LOVING GOD WHO WANTS US HEALED WHOLE AND SET FREE IN EVERY AREA OF OUR LIFE. - IN JESUS NAME. AMEN.

ZERO DAYS OF SHAME

*Y*es, Lord, zero days of Shame! We serve an amazing God. When I was a child, I experienced a lot of hurt and disappointment through the decisions of my parents. I was the eldest sibling and I took care of my younger siblings. I would cook for them, bathe them, and iron their clothes. I taught them how to read and write so I was just like a little young adult. As a child, I was very mature and had an enormous amount of responsibilities. I grew up in the projects, in fact, this was the longest time we were in one place. Then one day, there was a note put on our door that said that we had to move out. We were getting evicted; my mom went about her way and she went to work because she didn't know how to deal with it. She didn't face it head-on and she didn't get any boxes. We didn't pack up anything and one day the sheriff came and threw everything into the yard. People in the neighborhood were talking, and they called my mother's sisters and other family members. The family began to come around. At that moment, before they got there I sat on the steps and I began to pray and talk to God. I could feel the presence of Jesus all around me. I began to gain strength. I was ten years old, I had tears rolling down my face but, on the inside, I felt the presence of God. I knew that everything was going to be alright and that I had nothing to be ashamed of. It was in my childhood that I learned that in the midst of troubles, no matter what they may be, that you have nothing to be ashamed of. I found it to be so in the word of God: "hope maketh not ashamed because of Jesus Christ" (Romans 5: 5). Even after we were put out of our home in the projects, I still wanted to come back and play with my friend who lived next door to us. I decided I would go back to my now old neighborhood and play with her. I remember coming back to the neighborhood and kids were yelling, "didn't you get put out? Why you back over here?"

I held my little head high and I continued to move forward. I did what I wanted to do and then I went back to the place where we were now living.

Amid a powerful journey with my daughter, one day I began to look back at the things that I have experienced, and the things that God has brought me through. I began to recognize that God caused me to understand from a child that I had nothing to be ashamed of. No matter what my situation was because He was in control and that because of Jesus Christ, I could have hope and not be ashamed. What that means to me is that even though I'm going through trials and tribulations, because I got hope in Jesus Christ, I do not have to be ashamed. Everything is going to be alright.

What does that <u>mean</u> when you are going through troubling times? How does that <u>look</u> when you're going through? How does that <u>feel</u> when you're going through?

When you can see God's word showing up in your life it means everything! I made the decision that nothing was going to keep me from going to the house of the Lord. There were moments while sitting in church that people would be looking and staring, especially since our church started growing. Therefore, I started sitting in the back of the church with my daughter. After a visitor sat next to us and then got up and moved, they turned around from their new seat and continued to stare. I know that most people don't understand, that is why I wrote this book to help bring understanding because most people will only look at the outward symptoms. I never allowed people's responses to make me feel ashamed about my daughter. Even if she laughs, when no one else is laughing or she talks when no one else is talking. I learned to find ways to engage in conversation with her. I talked with her or just simply grabbed her by the hand, hugged her, and embraced her tightly so that she knows that she is loved and that she is not looked at differently by me regardless of how other people may look and stare, or what they may think or say. I never felt a day of shame. One blessed day, I had someone to say to me, "the way you love your daughter commands me to love your daughter". Another individual said to me, "when I see you with your daughter, I now know what love looks like", so I've gotten both sides.

DAILY DEVOTION:

Romans 5:5 King James Version (KJV) 5 And hope maketh not ashamed; because the love of God is shed abroad in our hearts by the Holy Ghost which is given unto us. King James Version (KJV) Isaiah 61:7-8 King James Version (KJV) 7 For your shame ye shall have double; and for confusion they shall rejoice in their portion: therefore, in their land they shall possess the double: everlasting joy shall be unto them.

Take a minute to reflect. Are you experiencing any shame for yourself or your loved one? What fear my you have about accepting your diagnosis or even your treatment plan? Don't give in to fear! BELIEVE the report of the Lord! (Use additional paper, if needed.)

_____

_____

_____

FINDING FULFILLMENT
DURING TOUGH TIMES

*L*ive your life as best you can despite your situation. I was given the strength to put one foot in front of the other through much prayer, fasting, and trusting God. He gave me strategies and insight. I truly understand what it means to say that the joy of the Lord is my strength. My whole life changed overnight. I had to learn how to talk to my daughter because initially, I was on eggshells. I didn't want to say anything that would upset her. Prior to the change, I never had to discipline her for anything. She never really raised her voice, she excelled naturally in school. As I reflect, I can remember noticing small changes. A lot was changing, and I began to realize that some of the changes that I was seeing were symptomatic to whatever was going on with her. Now, with the new medications, the more that I learned about the medications the more I had to be aware. I started to pay more attention to her behavior. I was praying to be able to distinguish between what she was dealing with internally versus the side effects of the medications.

Through it all, I never stopped going to church. In fact, I wanted to be to in church more and more. I prayed daily that God would bless us to be able to get to church safely. There were times that we would get to church, and I would have to turn around and leave because my daughter would have an episode. Sometimes she would scream out or yell and we would leave the church or go into another room. Other times, different church family leaders would walk around the church with her. It is such a blessing to see her sit through an entire service and there are days when she enjoys the praise and worship so much that it causes others around her to rejoice with her.

I truly understand when the word of God says, "take no thought for tomorrow, for tomorrow will take care of itself". There have been days when I have not been able to leave my apartment. By staying home with my daughter, I had to make a considerable amount of adjustments to rearrange my schedule to make sure she was safe and secure. By creating an environment that allows her to get help within our home, it helped to increase her independence. I knew that my daughter needed me more than ever. I am committed to being there for her. However, I still had to practice self-love and self-care. I learned to live my best life in the midst of my circumstances. It was my circumstances that I have seen God powerfully in our home and in my daughter's mind. I have felt the power and strength of God that gives me hope and courage to endure tough times.

I find myself in the word of God more and more. It has given me a greater anointing, and greater power to stand on the promises of God. To trust Him no matter what I see or hear. He said that "many are the afflictions of the righteous: but the Lord delivereth him out of them all" (Psalm 34:19). I see my daughter whole. I know healing is her portion. I speak positive words over her life. I know GOD is doing a new thing in her and it is happening NOW! He causes me to always move forward and to expect better and greater!

I always put safety first, the Lord has strengthened me to learn not to hold her to what happened that morning or whenever, but to look and see where she's at right now. I had to learn to live in the moment. I had to learn to assess where she was mentally and emotionally at the moment. Example, if we were going out to get ice cream, I had to assess her mood. By asking questions like, "are you calm now"? Can we still keep our plans? Otherwise, we would be confined to our home out of fear. God has not given us the spirit of fear, but of POWER, love and a sound mind. I can say that by making this shift in my mind, my faith increased which has helped me to live for NOW.

Therefore, I started my nonprofit organization called the *Art of Living No*w. The goal and prayer with this organization are to empower individuals and families to live their best life with what they have in their hands now. I stand on the word of God.

DAILY DEVOTION:

Psalm 118:17 King James Version (KJV) 17 I shall not die, but live, and declare the works of the Lord. Isaiah 54:17 New King James Version (NKJV) 17 No weapon formed against you shall prosper, And every tongue which rises against you in judgment You shall condemn. This is the heritage of the servants of the Lord, And their righteousness is from Me," Says the Lord. New King James Version (NKJV) Isaiah 43:18-19 King James Version (KJV) 18 Remember ye not the former things, neither consider the things of old. 19 Behold, I will do a new thing; now it shall spring forth; shall ye not know it? I will even make a way in the wilderness, and rivers in the desert. King James Version (KJV) Isaiah 59:19 King James Version (KJV) 19 So shall they fear the name of the Lord from the west, and his glory from the rising of the sun. When the enemy shall come in like a flood, the Spirit of the Lord shall lift up a standard against him. King James Version (KJV)

REFLECT AND JOURNAL YOUR THOUGHTS.

_____

_____

_____

_____

_____

_____

_____

_____

_____

_____

_____

_____

_____

_____

_____

_____

_____

_____

_____

_____

_____

_____

Debunking Mental Illness Stigmas

*D*ebunking the stigma of mental illness and changing our mindset when it comes to mental illness and disabilities. Let us start by looking at one another through a different lens. As I stated earlier, if an individual or their loved one has a physical ailment such as a broken arm they would not sit at home in silence and suffer, they will go out and seek the proper help. When it comes to mental illness, because culturally this has not been a topic of conversation in our communities, when it does occur, the first response for individuals, families, strangers and even providers are to fear the unknown. Fear can be very paralyzing, it causes you to shut down and not be responsive, caring, loving and supportive. The more you educate yourself and never lose sight of who your loved one is, you will be able to have a more positive mindset. Primarily, when you're dealing with the mind, there is a trauma or triggers related to the symptoms you are seeing. The brain is so complex, and everything functions through the mind. The brain goes into protection mode when an individual experiences something traumatic or stressful. It's important to seek proper help and to not be ashamed in the process of reaching out. As a society, we must change our mindset and response so that it's easier for those who need help to speak out. Why is it important to be informed? Think about the impact of CPR, and how it has saved so many lives. How many strangers have been helped by someone that took the time to learn a lifesaving skill? This is what we need to cultivate in our churches, communities and on our jobs. The more you learn, the sooner you can step up and give the support that is so desperately needed. We live and work in the same community. Together we can shut down the stigmas. The mere fact that I am writing this book right now indicates just how much all of this is happening. We all process things differently in life. This causes some people to have outward symptoms for something that is hurting them on the inside.

So how do we change the way society responds to mental illness? We must start by looking at each of the stigmas that are attached to mental illness. The biggest stigma that is attached to mental illness is the feeling of shame. We talked about shame earlier in the book, but it's necessary to revisit this topic because its prevalence is one of the main reasons why our community is underrepresented and suffering in silence. Shame causes isolation, and isolation can lead to several problems, including suicide. Isolation causes families to no longer to want to go out to engage with other people. They don't want to have any company over; they just stop doing the normal day-to-day things and find themselves completely consumed with managing their mental health or that of their loved one. I'm not saying that it's going to be easy to live your best life, however, you cannot allow any situation to cause you to be backed into a corner or cause you to be isolated and shut down. Yes, there will be moments where you may not be able to go anywhere because I have had many of those days where I was not able to go anywhere. I was confined to my home; I was in a position of figuring things out and readjusting my life I'm talking about weeks and even months of that. However, I did not disconnect myself from hope and believing that it was going to turn around. Shamefully, those going through this circumstance feel that other people, such as family and friends, will think something is wrong with them when they're trying to support their loved one. You may find yourself not inviting anyone over to your home or not wanting to go anywhere, and it's all because of shame. Accordingly, because of the word of God, I've been able to stand strong and not be ashamed. I know that I am loved and that my daughter is loved by God. He has kept a small group of the right people loving on us and supporting us!

Every opportunity that I can go somewhere to do something outside the home, I go for it. First, I assess our safety. Once I know we're safe to go out for a drive to grab some food from a restaurant or sit at the park, whatever it may be. With the help of God, I am living my best life in the midst of it all.

No one wakes up one day and says, "oh, I'm going to be the person that everybody stares at and everybody whispers about when I walk into a room".

Don't allow that to cause you to feel ashamed, don't allow that to cause you to shrink back in life. The simple thing is this, we're all being influenced by people one way or another whether it is negatively or positively. You must learn how to shut down the negativity and support your loved one. Do not allow any negative responses from anyone else to cause you to feel ashamed.

While you're supporting your loved one, they can feel what you feel because you're the closest one to them.

DAILY DEVOTION:

Say this Prayer:

"Lord, I thank you because the joy of the Lord is my strength. God, thank you because in your word you give me hope and you tell me that I have nothing to be ashamed of. No matter what my situation is you are in the midst of it. God, you bring me peace and you shine upon Me. Your Glory is upon me and God I thank you that hope maketh me not ashamed. Through your son Jesus Christ, I have hope for a better day. You said, "Many are the afflictions of the righteous: but the Lord delivereth him out of them all" and I choose to believe you. I choose to trust you and to stand in Faith, which gives me hope in you Lord! You also told us that you want us to live an abundant life. God, I am standing on your promises because you said your word shall not return void. It will do what you sent it out to do and that we are healed by Jesus` stripes. GOD, I know that you're able to do it in an instant, however, you choose to do it, God, I thank you for blessing me to walk victoriously through this process on this day. In Jesus mighty name I pray! Amen."

Isaiah 55:11 (KJV)

"So shall my word be that goeth forth out of my mouth: It shall not return void, but it shall prosper in the thing whereto I sent it."

REFLECT AND JOURNAL YOUR THOUGHTS.

_____

_____

_____

_____

_____

_____

_____

_____

_____

_____

_____

_____

_____

_____

_____

_____

_____

_____

_____

_____

Church, Healing
& Coping

*W*ow! When I think about church, I get a little choked up. If I can pause for just a moment and take a deep breath because I can sincerely and truly tell you that church is my lifeline. I have been going to church since I was an infant. My grandparents would take me to church with them as a little girl. It would start out early Saturday morning, they would be singing and cleaning the church and they would make sure the church grounds and the inside of the church were clean enough before Sunday morning services.

I remember, so vividly, that it was always dark when they finished because they were so engaged in praising God and just enjoying themselves while they were cleaning. They would break out into praise and worship songs. Then, they would go into prayer, and I just remember waking up with my grandparents putting me into the car. That was an amazing time for me in my younger life. Then, when I began to seek God for myself as a little girl, I would sit on the steps and just talk to God just like I can talk to an adult today. I would say things like, "God I know that you did not create me to just be born and live and just die". There must be more to this than just that". Then, one day an evangelist came into my community where I lived, and she began to talk about Jesus and everlasting life. I was around 7 years old and I got saved that day. I started walking to church with my siblings by myself. When we got baptized there were no adults there from my family. I knew I wanted to be saved. I wanted Jesus in my heart and in my life. I wanted to be baptized.

I wanted everlasting life. I was seeing so much at the time, at such an early age. I was a little girl when I was going to church with my grandparents. They lived in Georgia. I lived in a different state and as I began to grow up, I was always talking to God and trying to read the Bible; not really understanding it. At that time, I was always trying to read it and I remember walking around in my community just preaching not knowing exactly what I was saying. However, I had this little orange New Testament small Bible that you can find in a lot of different places and I would just be talking about the Lord. Those were seeds that were planted in me by my grandparents.

The church is so important to me; it means everything to me in a healthy way. When I say, "church", I'm not talking about the building. I mean my relationship with God, how I communicate with God, my posture towards God, my mindset when reading the word of God, and getting revelations from God. I have such a strong foundation and a strong relationship with God through His son Jesus Christ. My relationship with God has been the rock for me with everything concerning my daughter, from learning how to advocate for her with medications and the judiciary procedures through the court system. Without God, I would not have been able to walk this journey. Because of God, I am able to walk this journey one step at a time and one day at a time.

You may wonder how being in the church helped me with coping with the day to day struggles that I faced with my daughter. I can start by saying that I serve under an amazing and loving pastor, Dr. Riva Tims. She has been there from day one. When I didn't know what to do, the first thing I did was call on Jesus. The second thing I did was dial her number and she sent leaders over to my home. From there we started making decisions about what to do next. She called and checked on us almost every day. She could be out of town with an engagement to go on a talk show or be called away to preach at another church. She would be in the airport and the Lord would put us on her heart and she would just call us to see how we were doing. She has supported us financially too. This is how God shows up in your life, your relationship with God will give you favor with Him and mankind.

He causes others to step forward and be there for you. He will put you on the heart of others and cause them to move to help you. He will give them strategies on how to help you. It also speaks to her relationship with God and who she is as a person and how she loves God's people. Elder Michele serves as a leader in our church. She too would call me almost every day or text me. Each of these individuals spoke so much life into me at a time when everything had gone from 0 to 100. They also prayed for me endlessly along with other members and leaders from my church. This is how GOD shows up in your life. You just must recognize it!

Even if you're only able to raise your pinky finger to say, "I am still in the game"! Prayer is amazing. Prayer changes things. Prayer causes situations to shift in your favor. Prayer opens doors. Prayer brings Heaven down. Prayer shuts doors that should not be open.

I recall a situation where medication was recommended for my daughter and being that I am her advocate, I did my research on the medication and found that if she had taken the new medication, based on what was happening in her body physically with other medications, it could have caused some serious problems. What I had discovered about the medication was confirmed by three different individuals, some of which who were pharmacist, and they printed out the information for me and signed it. When I tried to present it to one of the doctors at the hospital it was rejected. One day, I went to visit my daughter with a family friend. I didn't know at the time that they were planning a hearing without my knowledge to try and have medication administered to my daughter without my consent and it was exposed. I was able to attend the hearing with an attorney and God gave me the favor I needed to claim victory.

I continue to be my daughter's advocate and represent her concerning her medications. The word that God gave me before the hearing was about Jehoshaphat. He was a king and there were armies that came against him and God sent a word by a prophet to tell him not to fear and to be still and know that God was in control and that He would not have to fight this battle. It was a reminder that the battle belonged to the Lord. God gave me that same word and He led me in the bible to read that passage. I did not have to open my mouth in that court hearing. I was able to get an attorney the morning of the hearing because I had just found out about the hearing. The attorney didn't get a chance to speak either, but GOD used her presence there in my favor and gave us the victory. In the end, that very same doctor wrote a powerful note about me in my daughter's discharge paper saying that my daughter was blessed to have a mom like me who was willing to fight for her and that I was a woman of integrity.

What I have found and what I've seen in the area of mental health and disabilities is that you're not just dealing with what your loved one is going through, but you're also having to navigate through varying entities and the different personalities of the doctors. The one thing that I found to be true, and I mean it took me back a bit, they treat families as if this was happening to us our entire lives and that this is all we knew. When in fact it was the total opposite. This was not happening to us our entire lives. It was a new experience and we were not having to deal with these types of medications. The strongest medications my daughter had taken up to this point was a Z-Pack for a cold. It could be your family's first day of really being impacted, your first week, your first month, or the first year; whatever the time frame may be, this is one of the things that really must change within our mental health professional community. In the beginning, because of how they would interact with my daughter I would often feel so unsure and fearful. I remember my daughter had a doctor's appointment; she had just been released from the hospital. The hospital had sent her records over to the doctor's office. Therefore, I was thinking that they were going to review her records and be prepared for us. I was hoping to gain some insight into what they read and to be ready to have a conversation about the state of her progression. Where she was at now in terms of her progress? Unfortunately, the doctor had never read the information that was sent over. She could not find the file and she had the audacity to say to me that she wouldn't have read it anyway even if she had it. She said that she needed to find out all the details from me right at that moment and the appointment was only for half an hour. Obviously, there was no way I could tell her everything about my daughter within such a limited time frame. During that appointment, my daughter had an outburst. This was early on and the doctor looked at me and said, "you know that I can have her put back in the hospital". I said to her, "why would you do that and why would you say that"? I informed the doctor that my daughter had just gotten home and that this was her first appointment as an outpatient. We were trying to find our way through this. I stated to her, "if she can't scream here with you where can she scream at"? I said to her, "You're supposed to help her through this and not just turn around say that to her because she screamed." My daughter left the room and she ran and got into the car. The good thing is that I didn't lock my car door that day, which is very unusual because I always locked my car door. I looked out the window and she was in the car and I finished my conversation with the doctor, and then I left. That day, I changed her doctor.

I never heard of the medical term "Baker Act". When my daughter experienced that it was scary for me, because I didn't know what to expect. It felt like they had all the control and I was just sitting and waiting for answers. Since the first time I heard that terminology, I've learned so much more. I understand so much more through prayer, support, and a lot of research. It took a lot of asking questions and seeking answers. I can tell you that I no longer walk on eggshells, something very significant and very major happened. Within that situation, I no longer walked on eggshells I prayed, and I talked to the Lord and I no longer walked in that fear!

GOD caused me to now walk in a place of confidence in my role of getting care for my daughter through this system of mental health and disabilities. From countless experiences of having to fill out paperwork and answer questions, working diligently to find the right medications, get the proper testing is done to help my daughter; I became more self-assured on how to navigate my way through the mental health care system.

I have had to pray about having individuals in my home to help my daughter. My prayer was to have the right people who will work to find resources and strategies to help her by communicating with the doctors.

We have experienced a lot, although I won't put every situation in this book, I will tell you that I am more than a conqueror through Christ Jesus. He causes us to always win and be victorious. I know that through this process God's healing, my family and I are fulfilling every promise and purpose that God has already planned for our lives for His GLORY. Through the process of healing and overcoming, we will help others along the way! There are loving men and women of God praying for my family right now!

Getting my daughter to church has been the most important thing in my life and I really mean that with every fiber of my being. I know when I get through those doors that we're going to be uplifted; we're going to be encouraged. This is a part of the healing process and breakthrough. I know that the presence of God is there. The word of God tells us to "assemble together", and when we all come together in unity there is power. We gather together to be in the presence of God to give Him Glory and to lift up the name of Jesus and to be restored in our mind, body, and soul, to have our mindset shifted, to be healed and made whole by the Spirit of the Lord God Almighty; never to leave the way that we came.

I know that God is omnipresent and that there is no distance in prayer. Some days, there has been a fight to get there, however, I can tell you that with the help of God through the power of God and through the love of God, His grace and His Mercy I am able to put one foot in front of the other. He gives me wisdom on how to gauge my daughter's mood so that we can be in the house of God. It has been a press on some days and a breeze on others. Laughter on some days and tears on other days, however through it all, I have learned to trust in the Lord on a greater level than ever before.

One of the things I had to come to realize through prayer and talking to the LORD, and again others praying with me and for me, is that NOTHING stops around you! Bill collectors still want their money. If you're working, you still have a job that you must be present at. The list goes on and on and on. I can say that I was blessed. I had a few people who paused with me on my journey. They were present in my life and gave my daughter and me the support and love that we needed. God ministered to me that the reason nothing can stop around me is that everything must progress forward around us as we are going through our journey. If He stopped everything around us in the state of where we are, what would God have to bring us forward to? What would you have to look forward to?

Remember when you're going through the fire, and you're faced with a challenge and you look around and it feels like no one is there and it feels like everyone is moving forward with their life, the day is going to come that God is going to redeem you forward into the things that he has for you because He allowed things to keep moving forward.

You can now be redeemed forward to all that God has for you to do. Remember God does not redeem you backward, He redeems you forward!

Momentum can flow in many directions. Momentum can flow backward or forward. God always causes you to go forward. Therefore, nothing can stop around us, and everything must go forward even though you may feel like you're spinning your wheels and you're on a treadmill or you are on a hamster wheel. Know that God will redeem you forward. The word of God says that "I shall live and not die that I shall declare the works of the LORD". What that simply means is that no matter what your state is ... just live. Even if living for you means that you spend the day in bed. Or if you push through and decide to get out of the bed that day, or even if it means that you've been in the house all week but today, you're deciding that you are going to go out to the mailbox. Whatever living is for you, live in the name of Jesus. Just live and Live NOW!

Always keep in mind that there are different times in your life where God will cause you to be set apart; not to harm you, but to give you hope and a future (read Jeremiah 29 and 11). We don't always know how that separation is going to come about. It can come through situations in our lives or sometimes just simply by God causing people who need to be removed from your life to be removed for you to move forward to where He is taking you in life for His Glory! You really don't know what you are made of until you are faced with a situation or challenge. Then, by faith, God shows up and shows you and others around you who He is! His power and love for you and those you love.

I love the book of Esther in the bible. Esther was a beautiful young woman. One day, her life went from zero to 100. I can relate to the sudden shift she endured. She too had to change her mindset to the will of God concerning her life; no matter the cost. God caused her to be set apart for such a time as this! She went on to save her people. You must read the entire book for yourself!

Chapter 4:13 Then Mordecai commanded to answer Esther, Think not with thyself that thou shalt escape in the king's house, more than all the Jews.

[14] For if thou altogether hold thy peace at this time, then shall there enlargement and deliverance arise to the Jews from another place; but thou and thy father's house shall be destroyed: and who knoweth whether thou art come to the kingdom for such a time as this?

[15] Then Esther bade them return Mordecai this answer,

[16] Go, gather together all the Jews that are present in Shushan, and fast ye for me, and neither eat nor drink three days, night or day: I also and my maidens will fast likewise; and so will I go in unto the king, which is not according to the law: and if I perish, I perish.

Isaiah 61:7-8 King James Version (KJV)

[7] For your shame ye shall have double; and for confusion, they shall rejoice in their portion: therefore, in their land they shall possess the double: everlasting joy shall be unto them.

[8] For I the Lord love judgment, I hate robbery for burnt offering; and I will direct their work in truth, and I will make an everlasting covenant with them.

Galatians 6:9 King James Version (KJV)

> [9] And let us not be weary in well doing: for in due season we shall reap, if we faint not.

Isaiah 40:31 King James Version (KJV)

> [31] But they that wait upon the Lord shall renew their strength; they shall mount up with wings as eagles; they shall run, and not be weary; and they shall walk, and not faint.

Daniel 11:32 KJV

> And such as do wickedly against the covenant shall he corrupt by flatteries: but the people that do know their God shall be strong and do exploits.

DAILY DEVOTIONS:

HE SAID HE WOULD NEVER LEAVE US NOR FORSAKE. HE HAS NEVER SEEN THE RIGHTEOUS FORSAKEN NOR IT'S SEED BEGGING FOR BREAD. Jehovah Rapha: The Lord, Our Healer. Our provider, our way maker, our everything!

> "Fight the good fight of the faith. Take hold of the eternal life to which you were called when you made your good confession in the presence of many witnesses." **1 Tim. 6:12**

"In all these things, we are more than conquerors through Him who loved us." **Rom. 8:37**

"Not by might nor by power, but by My Spirit,' says the Lord of hosts." **Zech. 4:6**

"Many are the afflictions of the righteous: but the Lord delivereth him out of them all." **Psalm 34:19**

"This is what the Lord says to you: 'Do not be afraid or discouraged because of this vast army. For the battle is not yours, but God's." **2 Chron. 20:15**

- When we belong to Christ, the enemy never has the final word over our lives. We are secure in God's hands.

- Press on – courageous and free – never held back by fear or defeat. The battle belongs to the Lord, and He has the final victory… IN CHRIST JESUS! AMEN

Psalm 91 King James Version (KJV)

^{91} He that dwelleth in the secret place of the most High shall abide under the shadow of the Almighty.

^{2} I will say of the Lord, He is my refuge and my fortress: my God; in him will I trust.

³ Surely he shall deliver thee from the snare of the fowler, and from the noisome pestilence.

⁴ He shall cover thee with his feathers, and under his wings shalt thou trust: his truth shall be thy shield and buckler.

⁵ Thou shalt not be afraid for the terror by night; nor for the arrow that flieth by day;

⁶ Nor for the pestilence that walketh in darkness; nor for the destruction that wasteth at noonday.

⁷ A thousand shall fall at thy side, and ten thousand at thy right hand; but it shall not come nigh thee.

⁸ Only with thine eyes shalt thou behold and see the reward of the wicked.

⁹ Because thou hast made the Lord, which is my refuge, even the most High, thy habitation;

¹⁰ There shall no evil befall thee, neither shall any plague come nigh thy dwelling.

¹¹ For he shall give his angels charge over thee, to keep thee in all thy ways.

¹² They shall bear thee up in their hands, lest thou dash thy foot against a stone.

[13] Thou shalt tread upon the lion and adder: the young lion and the dragon shalt thou trample under feet.

[14] Because he hath set his love upon me, therefore will I deliver him: I will set him on high, because he hath known my name.

[15] He shall call upon me, and I will answer him: I will be with him in trouble; I will deliver him, and honour him.

[16] With long life will I satisfy him, and shew him my salvation.

Psalm 23 King James Version (KJV)

[23] The Lord is my shepherd; I shall not want.

[2] He maketh me to lie down in green pastures: he leadeth me beside the still waters.

[3] He restoreth my soul: he leadeth me in the paths of righteousness for his name's sake.

[4] Yea, though I walk through the valley of the shadow of death, I will fear no evil: for thou art with me; thy rod and thy staff they comfort me.

[5] Thou preparest a table before me in the presence of mine enemies: thou anointest my head with oil; my cup runneth over.

[6] Surely goodness and mercy shall follow me all the days of my life: and I will dwell in the house of the Lord forever.

TENDER, LOVE & CARE...
WHAT EVERY HUMAN NEEDS

*W*hat does it mean to be a caregiver? According to the definition, a caregiver is a family member or paid helper who regularly looks after a child, or a sick, elderly, or disabled person. How do we define a disabled person? The Disability Discrimination Act (DDA) defines a disabled person as someone who has a physical or mental impairment that has a substantial and long-term adverse effect on his or her ability to carry out normal day-to-day activities. The DDA sets out the circumstances under which a person is 'disabled'. It's very important to understand the dynamics of what it means to be a caregiver. To care is caring for the wellbeing of someone else and even at times caring for them over caring for yourself. Giver means giving sacrificially of your time, yourself and even your finances. A caregiver is not something that happens overnight. If you had a chance to talk to most caregivers you will find that somewhere in their childhood, or teenage years, they were caring for their siblings or someone in their family. Maybe they were the ones having to care for all the pets that were in the family or the one all the neighborhood kids turned to for answers. Take me for example. I am my mom's eldest child and I cared for my younger siblings. I literally started cooking at the age of five. My mom was single and worked all the time. I recall standing in a chair over the stove because I made a decision that I no longer wanted to eat cold cereal. I wanted something hot for me, my brother, and sister to eat. So, I stood in the chair and I started cooking grits, eggs, and bacon. I remember the grease from the bacon popping and the hot grits popping but I did it! I did not give up and the meal came out great. I have been cooking ever since. My brother can still remember it too. I had watched my grandmother cook as a little girl and I was taking it in because I was always in the kitchen with her. I have a smile on my face as I'm writing this because the memories are so real and vivid. That's not the only thing I did, I taught my brother how to read, cleaned the house, and ironed the clothes. I did everything for my siblings. I didn't have much of a childhood. I was a very mature little girl and I took it very seriously about taking care of my siblings; I really looked after them. I even paid the bills for my mom and I monitored her bank account because I was getting money orders at a very young age. We lived in the projects and I would take the money orders to the housing authority and get my receipt and bring it back. Now when individuals would borrow money from my mom, I would be the one to collect the money back from them so that we could have food and the bills could continue to get paid.

Let us talk about self-care. Wow, life is so amazing. Now, listen to this: my grandparents had such a love for me they would send for me during the summer to spend time with them to get to know my family on my father's side. When I went to Georgia, I realized that something special was happening for me because I was going from the role of caring for my mom and my siblings to not having any adult responsibilities. It was only me and my grandparents, and the roles had reversed. I was now able to operate within the role of a child while having parental figures look after me. I can tell you with every fiber in my body that I knew that God was doing something awesome for me. I realized that what I was not getting at home, God was giving it to me through my grandparents. I realized that it was a time for me to just do nothing and just relax and enjoy myself. That's how I can tell you I know what it means to shift from being a caregiver to prioritizing self-care. However, on the same token, my cousin's in Georgia did not understand why

I didn't want to do anything. My grandparents had a working farm. I wanted to be in my grandfather's shadow; every move he made I wanted to be there. If he was in the hog-pen I wanted to be in the there too. If he was at a baseball game, I wanted to be at the baseball game too. I played checkers with him a lot. I did a lot of things with him and my grandmother and I mainly wanted to hang out with my Grandad. Every move he made; even when he sat in the chair to watch baseball. I had no clue what I was watching, but if I was sitting next to him it was okay. I would curl up in my grandparent's den and I started reading my aunt Gracie's love novels and some other books too. I was just enjoying the food! My grandmother cooked all my favorite foods: delicious caramel cakes, coconut cakes, pound cakes, and many other varieties of homemade foods. Like the fresh peas, okra and cream corn. She taught me how to eat it! It was amazing! The biggest point that I want to get across is that though I was a very young child, I understood the shift in the dynamics of what was happening in my life and I embraced it. My cousins did not understand why I didn't want to do anything, but my grandparents and I knew what I was going through. I knew the responsibility that was on me as a young girl. I knew all the things that I was doing, and once I got on that Greyhound bus for my grandparents to meet me and pick me up I knew that there was something different and special happening in my life. I was sure to fully embrace it!

What is self-care? For me as a caregiver, I always look forward to the day of my daughter's total healing and her flowing in the fullness of what God has for her and her independence. I speak and picture that as often as I possibly can in a very positive way. How do I find ways to care for myself? These days, it can be the simplest thing. Sometimes, I take myself out to dinner or to a movie. Sometimes, I just sit in my car and listen to my music a little longer or finish up a conversation with a friend before rushing back into the house. I love butterflies, so recently I took myself to a butterfly museum. I was treated to a spa day a few years ago. On another occasion, I was treated to a day at the nail salon and dinner. It was so nice, and I really appreciated that someone wanted to get me out of the house to do something just for me. This may not seem like much to others. However, for me, just the chance to do any of these things have been a blessing for me. I make it a priority to maintain my physical self-care, like getting my hair done at the salon. This is how God shows up in your life! I keep my hair done, I brush my teeth, I wear clean clothing, I wake up in my right mind, I can prepare my own meals, I read my bible, I pray for myself, for my family and for others. I shop and I enjoy eating out with friends. I love to dance to praise and worship music for the Lord! I love music. I want to travel and walk on beaches! I will do it ALL. I enjoy my quiet time too. I enjoy the days that I can sleep a little longer. I have dreams of getting married again! I desire that my next husband be someone who loves God more than he wants to be married; because then he will know how to love me right and cherish me like the jewel that I am.

Proverbs 3: 15-18 She is more precious than rubies; nothing you desire can compare with her. 16 Long life is in her right hand; in her left hand are riches and honor. 17 Her ways are pleasant ways, and all her paths are peace. 18 She is a tree of life to those who take hold of her; those who hold her fast will be blessed.

I am still learning, creating and growing in this process of hoping, believing and standing on the WORD of GOD by Faith!

Hebrews 11:1 King James Version (KJV)

Having a strong support system is so critical for anyone's wellbeing. For me, my grandparents played a significant role in helping me understand just how important it was to be there for those who you love, especially when they need you.

My grandparents were so significant in my childhood. Even as I sit here trying to express myself, I have to catch my breath because I don't quite know how to explain that

I knew as a child that my life at home with my mom wasn't adequate enough to sustain my growth. I needed to be loved and cared for as well. God gave me love and support through my grandparents. God was blessing me. I remember the sad day that my grandmother passed away and we all traveled to Georgia for her funeral. There was one day that all of the family was gathered together at my grandparents' home and an epiphany hit me like a ton of bricks. I realized when I looked around the room that this was the very first time in my entire life that I had seen my parents in the same room. No one knew what I was thinking, but I was talking to the Lord as I looked around with the understanding that this was a real moment for me. At that moment I realized that there is such a breakdown and tear down of the family unit that we don't really recognize it. It happens so often that it has become the norm. It becomes normal to see a single woman as head of households. That's not what God intended, that's not what he planned because the word of God says, "He who finds a wife finds a good thing and obtains favor from the Lord" (Proverbs 18:22). My grandparents were the example of love, support and really holding it down for the family. There was no mistaking that family was very important to them. Not just them but my grandparents' siblings also showed that same type of unity and love! They truly love the LORD AND FAMILY! Nothing or no one can take that from me it's such a big part of who I am. I experienced a lot of trauma myself as a young girl, my mother and her siblings were taken away from their mother, my grandmother, whom I never got the chance to meet. My grandmother's sister forced her to give up her children and she raised my mother and her siblings. The aunt who raised my mother and her siblings was very abusive towards them; both verbally and physically. I can remember my mother being whipped by her aunt as an adult with three children. My mother lived with her even after having me, my sister, and brother. Then one day after a disagreement between my mother and my aunt, my aunt kicked us out of her home.

One of my mother's sisters took us into her home to stay with her until my mom got her own apartment. We got our first apartment right across the way from my mother's sister. So, it began ... I was put in charge of my brother as my mom went to work. I was to keep the apartment clean, feed and watch my baby brother. My sister was not allowed to come with us, my mother's aunt took my sister from my mom. My mom's aunt raised my sister. My mother's aunt received welfare checks and food stamps for my mother and her siblings. Yet, she was continuing that same pattern with my baby sister. My mother feared her own aunt. During my childhood, I was given the task and roll that most elder children in the black community give their eldest child, and that task is to be in charge. Growing up, I often wondered about my grandmother on my mother's side of the family. The only thing I knew was that her name was Alice Toney. I always sat wondering what it must have felt like to have been forced away from her seven children. My only surviving uncle was an infant at the time and mom, along with her other siblings, who are all with the Lord now, were taken from their mother by her sister. My mom said she heard chatter from the grapevine that their mom may have settled in New York and that she had other children. My mother told me that my grandmother had tried to come back to get them, however, she was beaten so badly and sent away again. By this time, my grandfather was not with my grandmother anymore. I am not sure what happened there. By the time my maternal grandfather was involved in my life he was married to someone else. I was around my grandfather, but I wasn't close to him. Then I felt so sad for my mother too. She was a very giving person, anyone who knew her could ask her for anything and she would do it. Though that is a good quality to have, people will take advantage of it. I saw a lot of that which caused me to speak up about it at a very young age. For example, if my mom let friends borrow money or food stamps, I would be the one on the phone calling them up to have them return the money to mom so that we would have food and electricity. Back when I was growing up, it was the norm to leave young children home to care for the other children. I am not saying it was the right thing to do, that's what they did to survive. My mom has gone on to glory to be with LORD. She is not here to deny or confirm if what I am sharing is the truth or just my version of my childhood. However, what I can say is this that God always has a witness. There are still relatives living that were around to witness. One, in particular, intervened on my behalf on more than one occasion. As the years went by, my mom was very abusive towards me. She would slap me out of nowhere with no cause for it. Not that there is ever a cause for it in the first place. She would call me hurtful names. No matter what I did for my siblings it was never enough. Why do I share this with you now? Because during those abusive moments as a child I found myself asking GOD to help my mother because I felt that she had to be hurting from not having her mother with her for all those years. I felt so much love and sadness for my mother growing up. I witnessed her aunt beating her when I was a little girl. I remember saying to God when I grow up, I will never treat my children like this. Looking back in full clarity, I can see that God manifested His supernatural power over my life because I continued to feel love for my mother. I remember saying in my little prayers that "I forgive you, mom". My grandparents would arrange for me to spend summers with them as much as possible and my grandparents kept me in church. My grandmother always got on her knees before going to bed and said her prayers. I remember her being very quiet and never missing a night. Prayer is so powerful and real, when I wasn't with my grandparents and back home with my mother and siblings, I could always feel when my grandmother was praying for me. Even to this day I still feel her prayers because God said His word will not return void. Those same prayers are evident in my life today! I know it to be so because you're reading my story and I hope it helps you to break cycles in your family. As a child, I made a vow that I would not treat my children the way my mother treated me or the way her aunt treated her! Looking back, I realize that my mom did all she knew to do as it relates to her and how she processed her childhood. I am here to tell you that for me I knew as a child, I did not want the same for my children. I stand on the promises of God today to shut down the stigma of shame, fear, and isolation of mental illness and any type of disability. My prayers are that you release, forgive and let go to allow God to heal you and make you whole in every area of your life, your family and everyone connected to you. Men, you are important to the family unit! Stand up and take your rightful place in the Kingdom of God and in your families! Seek God for what that looks like at whatever state you're in!

Being a mother truly is an amazing gift and very humbling because I can tell you that it is driven by prayer for me. I love my children and grandbabies very deeply. When they are little you pray for them to be healthy and safe. You look forward to seeing them achieve every milestone. Things like learning to walk, feeding themselves, riding their bikes and the list goes on and on. One thing that remains consistent is praying for each one of them and you will see how your prayer life changes as they get older!

DAILY DEVOTION:

"For I am the LORD who heals you" - Exodus 15:26 NLT "He heals the brokenhearted and bandages their wounds" - Psalm 147:2 NLT "My wayward children ", says the LORD, "come back to me, and I will heal your wayward hearts." - Jeremiah 3:22 NLT "Then Jesus said, "Come to me, all of you who are weary and carry heavy burdens, and I will give you rest. Take my yoke upon you. Let me teach you, because I am humbled and gentle at heart, and you will find rest for your souls.""- Matthew 11:28-29 NLT

Prayer & Psychotropic Care

*N*ow, what a combination! First of all, I didn't even know what the word psychotropic[1] meant, what it was, what it entailed, in fact, it was nowhere on my radar for my life. Then one day I'm faced with trying to understand medications for my daughter, now I understood prayer in fact prayer is all that I knew. I knew the word of God, I lived my life, I went to church, I went to work. I took my children to school, I nurtured, loved and care for them as best as I could with the resources that I had.

Mental Health was nowhere on my mind for my children. I say that because there were times during my marriage I actually felt like my ex-husband showed signs of

---

[1] Psychotropic Medication- Any medication capable of affecting the mind, emotions and behavior. Some medications such as lithium, which may be used to treat depression, are psychotropic. Also called a psychodynamic medication.

depression and I attempted to talk to him about speaking to a minister or even a therapist. I did not know of any therapist myself, however, I was aware that we had 12 free visits to seek help through our Healthcare coverage. He said no, that nothing was wrong with him and that he did not need anyone telling him what to do.

He never sought help during our marriage. I prayed with and for him. It was difficult however I had to come to the realization that he was not going to go to therapy of any kind. I continued to pray daily and continuously and often. It is a part of my daily life. I don't see it as a routine. I see it as a necessity for my life.

Becoming familiar with psychotropic medications at first was very intimidating. As I stated earlier, once you read the side effects of the medications you are more informed about what to look out for and what to pray for. There is a lot of trial and error. Starting over with new medications, continuous blood work and researching each new medication when they want to make any changes.

The only thing that has gotten me through this process is my prayer life, my relationship with God and staying in the word of God! I had to trust God on a whole new level that I had not seen before. Researching the medications and getting the answers I need to make the best decisions for my daughter's care. Yes, prayer has gotten me through the process of understanding psychotropic medications while still doing research and learning. My faith increased to a level it had not been before and it took prayer not just researching the medications. Me praying for myself and most definitely others praying for me and my family, my pastor, my family, our intercessors' team in my church and friends. I can tell you that through prayer and the WORD OF GOD my mindset changed and I no longer walk in fear when it comes to the medications. I am praying and believing God for total healing for my daughter, she shall recover it All!

Through prayer, I have hope in Christ JESUS that my daughter shall do ALL that she is purposed to do! Always stand by faith never come in agreement with the diagnoses or the symptoms. Follow the instructions given to you by the doctor and hold on for a better tomorrow. I still pray about every medication choice and my daughter's overall care. Mentally, physically, spiritually and socially as well! When it comes to the medications even my daughter's mindset has changed. I remember when she first started taking medication for the challenges that she was now facing it was very difficult for her because for her that meant something was wrong with her and it felt like it was all happening so fast. Growing up the strongest medication she had taken at that point in her young beautiful life was a

Z Pack for a cold. It is still a process and we take it one day at a time. My daughter is an amazing, loving, giving, caring, very talented humble young woman who loves JESUS, she loves God and His people!

CULTIVATING A MINDSET OF GRATITUDE

*T*he importance of cultivating a mindset of gratitude, This is important because when you have a mindset of gratitude which is being thankful it is impossible to have a negative mindset. For example, no matter what your situation is, if you look for the positive and focus on that, you will begin to have a mindset of gratitude and there is no room for negativity. Your mood will shift and you can feel yourself smiling. Your outlook on your situation will begin to change, it can be the smallest things that can cause you to find gratitude in your situation. One morning I got dressed to go meet my clients. I got into my car and backed out of my garage. Something felt different and I heard this sound coming from my tires. I got out of my car and I had a flat tire. Now I could have gotten upset because I was scheduled to meet clients however instead, I remained calm and immediately I was so thankful and grateful that the flat tire happened while my car was parked at home in my garage. I have roadside service that will come to me. I am safe in front of my driveway. This did not happen while I was driving. I contribute all of this to prayer and my mindset to first remain calm and immediately started thinking about all the things I have to be grateful and thankful for and not focus on all of the negatives thoughts that will try to rise up. You may say oh my situation is worse than getting a flat tire and trust me I understand that part too. However, I used an uncomplicated example for two reasons. First to get to you thinking about how to apply this to your everyday living and second there are individuals who have exploded for less and then take it out on others around them. To finish my example. I called my clients and they were very understanding and in fact, they offered to come to pick me up in their car for our scheduled appointment. We had a great day and an amazing outcome!

What is the benefit of cultivating a mindset of gratitude? There are health benefits decrease in stress and disease. Healthier Mindset means a healthier you and a healthier community as a whole. Having a mindset of gratitude will give you a stronger immune system, fewer aches, and pain, lower your blood pressure, more rested.

With social media on the rise having a mindset of gratitude will also increase your social life, more outgoing, compassionate, forgiving and it helps to illuminate you from feeling lonely and isolated. Psychologically your mindset shifts in a more positive direction and your more alert alive and full of joy. People around you can see it and feel it as well. Will there be days you just want to be alone, yes most definitely! However, don't gravitate to that when issues arise it will only pull you into isolation and shift your mind into negativity. If you see someone struggling in this area find a positive way to share with them ways of getting help.

Throughout the Bible, you will find passages of Scripture that teaches you about gratitude and being thankful. Cultivating a mindset of gratitude is something you have to choose daily. I hope you find comfort in the scriptures listed below. Remember you have the power to choose how you're going to respond to a situation, a person or a doctor's report. You can replace a negative thought or response with positivity!

"Do not be anxious for anything, but in everything by prayer and supplication with thanksgiving let your requests be made known to God." **Phil 4:6**

"Bless the Lord, O my soul, and all that is within me, bless his holy name! Bless the Lord, O my soul, and forget not all his benefits, who forgives all your iniquity, who heals all your diseases, who redeems your life from the pit, who crowns you with steadfast love and mercy, who satisfies you with good so that your youth is renewed like the eagle's." **Ps. 103:1-5**

"Give thanks in all circumstances; for this is the will of God in Christ Jesus for you." **1 Thess. 5:18**

"Oh give thanks to the Lord, for he is good, for his steadfast love endures forever!" **Ps. 107:1**

"Giving thanks always and for everything to God the Father in the name of our Lord Jesus Christ," **Eph. 5:20**

"The Lord is my strength and my shield; My heart trusts in Him, and I am helped; Therefore, my heart exults, And with my song I shall thank Him." **Ps. 28:7**

"I will praise the name of God with song, and shall magnify Him with thanksgiving." **Ps. 69:30**

"Give thanks to the Lord, for he is good, for his steadfast love endures forever. Give thanks to the God of gods, for his steadfast love endures forever. Give thanks to the Lord of lords, for his steadfast love endures forever; to him who alone does great wonders, for his steadfast love endures forever; to him who by understanding made the heavens, for his steadfast love endures forever; ..." **Ps. 136:1-5**

"Therefore, since we are receiving a kingdom that cannot be shaken, let us be thankful, and so worship God acceptably with reverence and awe, for our "God is a consuming fire." **Heb. 12:28-29**

"Thanks be to God for his inexpressible gift!"
2 Cor. 9:15

"We give thanks to you, Lord God Almighty, the One who is and who was, because you have taken your great power and have begun to reign."
Rev. 11:17

"Amen! Praise and glory and wisdom and thanks and honor and power and strength be to our God forever and ever. Amen!" **Rev. 7:12**

A PRAYER OF GRATITUDE:

Thank you, Heavenly Father, for blessing me to wake up to a brand-new day that I've never seen before. Thank you, Heavenly Father, for New Beginnings in Christ Jesus. God, I thank you for your protection. I thank you for providing, and for always making a way out of no way. I thank you for sending Divine connections and providing resources for me, my family and others around me. I thank you, Lord, for my daily bread. I thank you for your love and your favor I thank you for giving me a clear direction. I thank you for peace in my home and peace in my mind. Thank you for your HEALING power in my life, my children, my grandchildren, and my family. I thank you for always causing me to be victorious in Christ Jesus! Amen!

Grateful

[**greyt**-f*uh*l]

Adjective

Warmly or deeply appreciative of kindness or benefits received; thankful: *I am grateful to you for your help.* expressing or actuated by gratitude: *a grateful letter.* pleasing to the mind or senses; agreeable or welcome; refreshing: *a grateful breeze.*

EXTENDING GRACE

The importance of extending "Grace". Something as simple as an act of kindness to someone in need can change their outlook on life. Not everyone is looking for material things or big over the top gestures. You will be surprised how a sincere heartfelt word can shift the course of someone's life. Use your Words wisely: Be kind and gentle in what you say and how you say it. You've all heard this before "words don't hurt well that's not true. Words have power and they do hurt. Let's take a look at emotional pain. Pain can come from the words that we say to one another. Then emotional pain if not dealt with can and will cause physical pain and illnesses. Think about moments you were doing great and you set out on your day, someone calls you and during the conversation they something subtle. You hang up the phone and now you're feeling some kind of way, now you're trying to figure out what happened? Why I am feeling this way? Then you trace it back to that conversation. "WORDS" Here's what the Word of GOD has to say about that.

> 1."A gentle answer turns away wrath, But a harsh word stirs up anger." **Proverbs 15**

> 2. Let your conversation be always full of grace, seasoned with salt, so that you may know how to answer everyone. **Colossians 4:6**

> 3. Death and life are in the power of the tongue: and they that love it shall eat the fruit thereof. **Proverbs 18:21**

Clearly, you can see through these passages of Scriptures that words have power and how will you choose to use that power? Now if you're on the receiving end of someone not extending Grace but instead negativity. You too have the power to not RECIEVE it! Do not except any negativity in your life no matter what or who. Forgive them and begin speaking life into yourself, write it down, speak it out loud, record yourself speaking positive words about your life and play it back. This is reinforcement for encouragement. The Word commands us to encourage ourselves sometimes and when you feel like you can't. Playback some of your recordings or read a page or two from your journal of positive thinking and affirmations you have written down. It's very important to write as much as possible. It clears your mind, helps you to set things in order, helps you to remember things better, organize your thoughts, helps to give you clear direction and most of ALL in those times of needing GRACE in your life you have something to fall back on for encouragement to lift you up and keep you moving forward instead of going backward. Momentum is always in motion it's either going backward or forward you get to choose which direction you want to move in, choose moving forward in spite of! I encourage you to stay in the Word of GOD!

> And the Lord answered me and said: "Write the vision and make it plain upon tablets, that he may run that readeth it. **Habakkuk 2:2**

My prayer for you: Thank you GOD that Grace abounds! I pray for each and every person reading this, GOD I pray that you will shower them with your love, Grace, and mercies to move forward! To stay focused and to remain calm and trust the process. To look to you GOD the author and finisher of their Faith. I pray restoration, peace, forgiveness, love, wholeness, FAVOR and HEALING NOW LORD IN JESUS MIGHTY NAME!

MIND OVER MATTER

Isaiah 38 King James Version (KJV)

[38] In those days was Hezekiah sick unto death. And Isaiah the prophet, the son of Amoz came unto him, and said unto him, thus saith the LORD, set thine house in order: for thou shalt die, and not live.

[2] Then Hezekiah turned his face toward the wall, and prayed unto the LORD,

[3] And said, remember now, O LORD, I beseech thee, how I have walked before thee in truth and with a perfect heart, and have done that which is good in thy sight. And Hezekiah wept sore.

[4] Then came the word of the LORD to Isaiah, saying,

[5] Go, and say to Hezekiah, thus saith the LORD, the God of David thy father, I have heard thy prayer, I have seen thy tears: behold, I will add unto thy days fifteen years.

^{6.} And I will deliver thee and this city out of the hand of the king of Assyria: and I will defend this city.

^{7.} And this shall be a sign unto thee from the LORD, that the LORD will do this thing that he hath spoken;

1. The first thing that we will look at is that Hezekiah did not mix any words with the prophet. Also, he did not come into agreement with what was spoken by the prophet.

2. Note that Isaiah and King Hezekiah knew each other, and King Hezekiah knew that Isaiah was a true prophet of GOD. Even in knowing all of that he put **"MIND OVER MATTER"** and turned his face to the wall and began to cry out to GOD for himself. Hezekiah did not waste any time, nor did he try to call out to 10 other people. He did not get on "Facebook", nor did he send out a 'telegram' or wait a minute 'Instagram' He went straight to GOD!

3. It wasn't that what the prophet said was not factual because it was, it was evident through the physical pain, hurt, shame and uncertainty that King Hezekiah was experiencing and on top of that a true prophet comes

into a room to deliver a message from GOD. Hezekiah still turned his head to the wall, and he began to cry out to GOD for himself! He spoke in detail to GOD WITHOUT SHAME OR HESITATION!

4.   ONLY GOD CAN CHANGE HIS OWN WORDS!

5.   GOD IMMEDIATELY sent Isaiah back to tell Hezekiah, I hear your cry and I see your tears and GOD added 15 more years to Hezekiah's life! Only GOD! But GOD!!!!

In closing

1.   How do you relate this to your life today?

A.   What are some examples – doctor's report

Some of you or a loved one may have gotten a bad doctor's report. Do not come in agreement with it. There may be steps or instructions from the physician/doctor that may have to be followed, however, you must apply "MIND OVER MATTER" turn your face to the wall and open your mouth and cry out to GOD for yourself! IN JESUS MIGHTY NAME!!! AMEN

Reference scripture: Isaiah 59: 19 [KJV]

> ^{19.} So shall they fear the name of the LORD from the west, and his glory from the rising of the sun. When the enemy shall come in like a flood, the Spirit of the LORD shall lift a standard against him.

B. How do I apply **"MIND OVER MATTER"** to my daily life?

1. Through reading and listening to the LIVING WORD OF GOD

2. Through the leading and guiding of the HOLY SPIRIT

3. Through prayer and calling on the name JESUS

4. Crying out to GOD

5. Through Fasting

6. Believing beyond what you're feeling and seeing in front of you, see beyond what you see

7. Standing in FAITH every man was given a measure of faith! Stand!

Reference scripture: Psalm 34:19 – Many are the afflictions of the righteous: but the LORD delivered him out of them all.

Romans 8:18-19 – 18. For reckon that the suffering of this present time are not worthy to be compared with the glory which shall be revealed in us. 19. For the earnest expectation of this creature waited for the manifestation of the sons of GOD.

Isaiah 54:17 – 17. No weapon that is formed against thee shall prosper; and every tongue that shall rise against thee in judgment thou shalt condemn. This is the heritage of the servants of the LORD, and their righteousness is of me, saith the LORD.

Isaiah 43:18-19 – 18. Remembering ye not the former things, neither consider the things of old. 19. Behold, I will do a new thing; now it shall spring forth; shall ye not know it? I will even make a way in the wilderness, and rivers in the desert.

Jeremiah 29:11- 11. For I know the thoughts that I think towards you, saith the LORD, thoughts of peace, and not of evil, to give you an expected end.

Psalm 91: 1 – 1. He that dwelleth in the secret place of the most HIGH shall abide under the shadow of the Almighty.

A Call for Salvation

If you don't know Jesus and would like to know more about His love and what it means to be saved and receive salvation now. Please repeat these words

Prayer for Salvation

"Father GOD forgive me of my sins I don't want to be like this anymore. I want to serve you GOD and I accept Jesus into my heart now LORD. I accept JESUS AS MY LORD. I confess my sins and ask for forgiveness. You are my GOD and I am your child and servant. Have your way LORD in my life and I will serve you all the days of my life! Fill me with your precious Holy Spirit now, LORD. With the evidence of speaking in tongues, In Jesus` name! Amen.

Romans: 5:5 Hope makes not ashamed in Christ Jesus, Amen!

HEARTFELT DEDICATIONS, REFLECTIONS AND POEMS FOR MY DARLING DAUGHTER ASHLEE

To Ashlee from your big Brother:

"It has been my philosophy of life that difficulties vanish when faced boldly." -**Isaac Asimov**

"Times of great calamity and confusion have ever been productive of the greatest minds. The purest ore is produced from the hottest furnace, and the brightest thunderbolt is elicited from the darkest storm." -**Charles Caleb Colton**

"The gem cannot be polished without friction, nor man be perfected without trials." -**Danish Proverb**

Throughout your life, I have watched you grow into an intelligent, witty, and charming young lady. You have accomplished many things thus far, with much more to come. Of all your successes I have never been prouder and honored to call you my sister, than watching you power through life's challenges. Although it may not be verbalized every day, your progress shows. You have been blessed by God in the name of Jesus to stand in the midst of it ALL.

Take a moment to absorb that fact. Take another to understand the magnitude of powering through life's trials with the ability to look back and know that you are still here. Now, look forward towards the future, for it is waiting patiently for you to conquer it. You have always been that lightening escaping from the storm and that diamond unbound from tempered coal. There are not enough words to express a quantification of your abilities and possibilities. Nor are there enough to express my love as your brother. I only hope that these will suffice.

I love you; Ashlee and God Bless you!

-**Leon**

Dedication Letter

To Ashlee from your big Sister:

What a blessing it is to have you as my younger sister. Witnessing your growth has been such a gift. Through any obstacle placed in your life, you've proven that you are becoming a stronger, more fearless, and beautiful every day. Your struggles are not in vain. You have a divine purpose.

You have a long and fulfilling life ahead of you. Continue to have faith in your abilities and your strength to overcome anything, and you will. Continue to lean on your divine power of being a woman through the good and bad and The Most High will never steer you wrong.

The smallest light can brighten the darkest cave. Continue to be the light of awareness for mental health. I know you will enlighten this world so that future generations will have a brighter future and feel safe to express their truth. I am proud of you, my remarkable sister.

Always and forever.

Shontae`

Perception and Truth
By Ashlee McLoyd

So many points of view. Everyone talking off of each other's verbal cues. Confusing the natural homeostasis of everyday conversations

With classic scenarios, does anyone know how it really goes? Two sides and the truth?

No, I say just a justification for the uncouth.

All the world's a stage, but what a rarity it would be if everyone was on the same page.

Perception and truth are seldom one and the same. It can confuse a harlot for the likes of a great dame. A harvest you are bound to reap

By the thoughts that you choose to speak.

Images and ideas are built into minds. Fantasies of so many different kinds. It is all in the way you perceive, for some these ideas are the hope to which they cleave.

Published in the 8th grade

BREATHE
BY ASHLEE MCLOYD

I want to breathe.

We walk around working

ourselves into the ground.

Smiles, laughter, but

What is the heart of the world after?

Dreams, maybe goals?

Yet for so many there is still a hole.

The heart craves.

While the world raves.

And to what end?

Where is the world headed?

Promiscuity, violence and drugs.

Freedom as fleeting as friendly hugs.

We push while we heave.

However, the answer is incredibly simple.

We just want to breathe.

PREVALENCE
OF MENTAL ILLNESS

Source - "NAMI"

- Approximately 1 in 5 adults in the U.S. (46.6 million) experiences mental illness in a given year.1

- Approximately 1 in 25 adults in the U.S. (11.2 million) experiences a serious mental illness in a given year that substantially interferes with or limits one or more major life activities.2

- Approximately 1 in 5 youth aged 13–18 (21.4%) experiences a severe mental disorder at some point during their life. For children aged 8–15, the estimate is 13%.3

- 1.1% of adults in the U.S. live with schizophrenia.4

- 2.6% of adults in the U.S. live with bipolar disorder.5

- 6.9% of adults in the U.S.—16 million—had at least one major depressive episode in the past year.6

- 18.1% of adults in the U.S. experienced an anxiety disorder such as posttraumatic stress disorder, obsessive-compulsive disorder, and specific phobias.7

- Among the 20.2 million adults in the U.S. who experienced a substance use disorder, 50.5%—10.2 million adults—had a co-occurring mental illness.8

Social Stats

- An estimated 26% of homeless adults staying in shelters live with serious mental illness and an estimated 46% live with severe mental illness and/or substance use disorders.9

- Approximately 20% of state prisoners and 21% of local jail prisoners have "a recent history" of a mental health condition.10

- 70% of youth in juvenile justice systems have at least one mental health condition and at least 20% live with a serious mental illness.11

- Only 41% of adults in the U.S. with a mental health condition received mental health services in the past year. Among adults with a serious mental illness, 62.9% received mental health services in the past year.8

- Just over half (50.6%) of children with a mental health condition aged 8-15 received mental health services in the previous year.12

- African Americans and Hispanic Americans each use mental health services at about one-half the rate of Caucasian Americans and Asian Americans at about one-third the rate.13

- Half of all chronic mental illness begins by age 14; three-quarters by age 24. Despite effective treatment, there are long delays—sometimes decades—between the first appearance of symptoms and when people get help.14

Consequences of Lack of Treatment

- Serious mental illness costs America $193.2 billion in lost earnings per year.15

- Mood disorders, including major depression, dysthymic disorder, and bipolar disorder, are the third most common cause of hospitalization in the U.S. for both youth and adults aged 18–44.16

- Individuals living with serious mental illness face an increased risk of having chronic medical conditions.17 Adults in the U.S. living with serious mental illness die on average 25 years earlier than others, largely due to treatable medical conditions.18

- Over one-third (37%) of students with a mental health condition age 14–21 and older who are served by special education drop out—the highest dropout rate of any disability group.19

- Suicide is the 10th leading cause of death in the U.S. and the 2nd leading cause of death for people aged 10–34.20

- More than 90% of people who die by suicide show symptoms of a mental health condition.21

- Each day an estimated 18-22 veterans die by suicide.22

CITATIONS

1. Any Mental Illness (AMI) Among Adults. (n.d.).
    Retrieved May 1, 2019,
    from https://www.nimh.nih.gov/health/statistics/
    mental-illness.shtml#part_154785

2. Serious Mental Illness (SMI) Among Adults. (n.d.).
    Retrieved May 1, 2019,
    from https://www.nimh.nih.gov/health/statistics/
    mental-illness.shtml#part_154788

3. Any Disorder Among Children. (n.d.) Retrieved
    January 16, 2015,
    from http://www.nimh.nih.gov/health/statistics/pr
    evalence/any-disorder-among-children.shtml

4. Schizophrenia. (n.d.). Retrieved January 16, 2015,
    from http://www.nimh.nih.gov/health/statistics/pr
    evalence/schizophrenia.shtml

5. Bipolar Disorder Among Adults. (n.d.). Retrieved
    January 16, 2015,
    from http://www.nimh.nih.gov/health/statistics/pr
    evalence/bipolar-disorder-among-adults.shtml

6. Major Depression Among Adults. (n.d.). Retrieved
    January 16, 2015,

from http://www.nimh.nih.gov/health/statistics/pr evalence/major-depression-among-adults.shtml

7.   Any Anxiety Disorder Among Adults. (n.d.). Retrieved January 16, 2015, from http://www.nimh.nih.gov/health/statistics/pr evalence/any-anxiety-disorder-among-adults.shtml

8.   Substance Abuse and Mental Health Services Administration, *Results from the 2014 National Survey on Drug Use and Health: Mental Health Findings*, NSDUH Series H-50, HHS Publication No. (SMA) 15-4927. Rockville, MD: Substance Abuse and Mental Health Services Administration. (2015). Retrieved October 27, 2015 from http://www.samhsa.gov/data/sites/default/fi les/NSDUH-FRR1-2014/NSDUH-FRR1-2014.pdf

9.   U.S. Department of Housing and Urban Development, Office of Community Planning and Development. (2011). *The 2010 Annual Homeless Assessment Report to Congress.* Retrieved January 16, 2015, from https://www.hudexchange.info/resources/do cuments/2010HomelessAssessmentReport.pdf

10.   Glaze, L.E. & James, D.J. (2006). *Mental Health Problems of Prison and Jail Inmates.*Bureau of Justice Statistics Special Report. U.S. Department of Justice, Office of Justice Programs Washington, D.C. Retrieved March 5, 2013,

from http://bjs.ojp.usdoj.gov/content/pub/pdf/m
hppji.pdf

11. National Center for Mental Health and Juvenile
Justice. (2007). *Blueprint for Change: A Comprehensive
Model for the Identification and Treatment of Youth with
Mental Health Needs in Contact with the Juvenile Justice
System.* Delmar, N.Y: Skowyra, K.R. & Cocozza, J.J.
Retrieved January 16, 2015,
from http://www.ncmhjj.com/wp-
content/uploads/2013/07/2007_Blueprint-for-
Change-Full-Report.pdf

12. Use of Mental Health Services and Treatment
Among Children. (n.d.). Retrieved January 16, 2015,
from http://www.nimh.nih.gov/health/statistics/pr
evalence/use-of-mental-health-services-and-
treatment-among-children.shtml

13. Substance Abuse and Mental Health Services
Administration, *Racial/Ethnic Differences in Mental
Health Service Use among Adults.* HHS Publication No.
SMA-15-4906. Rockville, MD: Substance Abuse and
Mental Health Services Administration, 2015.
Retrieved July 2017,
from https://www.samhsa.gov/data/sites/default/f
iles/MHServicesUseAmongAdults/MHServicesUse
AmongAdults.pdf.

14. Kessler, R.C., et al. (2005). Prevalence, Severity, and
Comorbidity of 12-Month DSM-IV Disorders in the
National Comorbidity Survey Replication. *Archives of*

General Psychiatry, *62*(6), 593–602. Retrieved January 16, 2015,

from http://archpsyc.jamanetwork.com/article.aspx?articleid=208671

15. Insel, T.R. (2008). Assessing the Economic Costs of Serious Mental Illness. The American Journal of Psychiatry. 165(6), 663-665

16. Agency for Healthcare Research and Quality, The Department of Health & Human Services. (2009). *HCUP Facts and Figures: Statistics on Hospital-based Care in the United States, 2009*. Retrieved January 16, 2015, from http://www.hcup-us.ahrq.gov/reports/factsandfigures/2009/pdfs/FF_report_2009.pdf

17. Colton, C.W. & Manderscheid, R.W. (2006). Congruencies in Increased Mortality Rates, Years of Potential Life Lost, and Causes of Death Among Public Mental Health Clients in Eight States. *Preventing Chronic Disease: Public Health Research, Practice and Policy*, *3*(2), 1–14. Retrieved January 16, 2015,

from http://www.ncbi.nlm.nih.gov/pmc/articles/PMC1563985/

18. National Association of State Mental Health Program Directors Council. (2006). *Morbidity and Mortality in People with Serious Mental Illness.* Alexandria, VA: Parks, J., et al. Retrieved January 16, 2015

from http://www.nasmhpd.org/docs/publications/
MDCdocs/Mortality%20and%20Morbidity%20Fina
l%20Report%208.18.08.pdf

19. U.S. Department of Education. (2014). *35th Annual Report to Congress on the Implementation of the Individuals with Disabilities Education Act, 2013*. Washington, DC: U.S. Department of Education. Retrieved January 16, 2015,
from http://www2.ed.gov/about/reports/annual/o
sep/2013/parts-b-c/35th-idea-arc.pdf

20. National Institutes of Mental Health (2018). "Suicide." Retrieved December 6, 2018,
from https://www.nimh.nih.gov/health/statistics/s
uicide.shtml

21. Isometsa, E.T., (2001). Psychological Autopsy Studies - A Review. *European Psychiatry,*16(7), 379-85. Retrieved December 6, 2018, from
https://www.ncbi.nlm.nih.gov/pubmed/11728849

22. U.S. Department of Veteran Affairs Mental Health Services Suicide Prevention Program. (2012). *Suicide Data Report, 2012*. Kemp, J. & Bossarte, R. Retrieved January 16, 2015,
from http://www.va.gov/opa/docs/Suicide-Data-
Report-2012-final.pdf

23. Lipscomb, J. (2017, June 09). Retrieved from Miami New Times: https://www.miamin Lipscomb, J. (2017, June 09). Retrieved from Miami New Times: https://www.miaminewtimes.com/news/audit-says-

state-mental-hospitals-are-understaffed-and-dont-meet-fire-code-9406198 ewtimes.com/news/audit-says-state-mental-hospitals-are-understaffed-and-dont-meet-fire-code-9406198

RESOURCES

NAMI
3803 N. Fairfax Drive,
Suite 100
Arlington, VA 22203
Main: **703-524-7600**
Member Services
888-999-6264
Helpline
800-950-6264

NAMI PROGRAMS
NAMI Basics
NAMI Connection
NAMI Ending the Silence
NAMI Family Support Group
NAMI Family-to-Family
NAMI Homefront
NAMI In Our Own Voice
NAMI Peer-to-Peer
NAMI Parents & Teachers as Allies
NAMI Provider Education
MENTAL ILLNESS
ADHD
Anxiety Disorders
Bipolar Disorder

Borderline Personality Disorder
Depression
Dissociative Disorders
Eating Disorders
Obsessive-Compulsive Disorder
Posttraumatic Stress Disorder
Schizoaffective Disorder
Schizophrenia
RELATED CONDITIONS
Anosognosia
Dual Diagnosis
Psychosis
Self-harm
Sleep Disorders
Suicide

Mental Health Association of Central
1525 E Robinson St, Orlando, FL 32801
1 407-898-0110
We provide Suicide Prevention, Anxiety & Depression
Support, Guardian Advocates, & other Mental Health
Services ... Please check your local listing for Mental
Health Association - MHA

You're not alone. Confidential help is available for free.
National Suicide Prevention Lifeline
Call **1-800-273-8255**
Available 24 hours every day

You're not alone. Confidential help is available for free.
National Suicide Prevention Lifeline
Call **1-800-273-8255**
Available 24 hours everyday

We can all help prevent suicide. The Lifeline provides 24/7, free and confidential support for people in distress, prevention and crisis resources for you or your loved ones, and best practice.

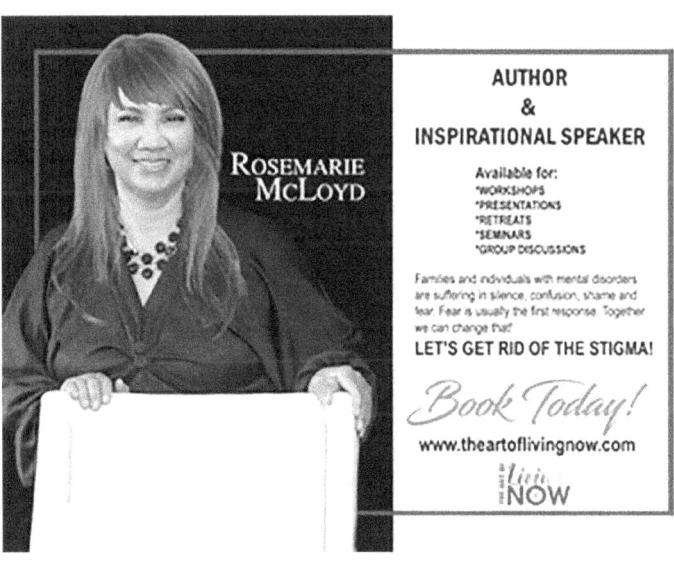

Rosemarie McCoy McLoyd
President, Founder and CEO
The Art Of Living Now, Inc. – Nonprofit
Http://www.theartoflivingnow.com
Admin@theartoflivingnow.com
Rosemariemcloyd@theartoflivingnow.com

.